The Body-clock Diet

Dr Alan Maryon Davis

D1079106

Network Books

About the Author

Dr Alan Maryon Davis is one of this country's best-known media doctors, familiar to millions from his many TV and radio interviews and such peak-time series as BBC 1's *Bodymatters* and *The BBC Diet Programme*. He is the health advisor for *Woman* magazine and the author of eight popular books on health including the bestselling *Diet 2000*. In his 'spare time' he is a public health doctor in south London and a member of the humorous singing group *Instant Sunshine*.

Network Books is an imprint of BBC Books,
a division of BBC Worldwide Publishing,
Woodlands, 80 Wood Lane, London W12 0TT

First published 1996
Reprinted 1996

ISBN 0 563 37159 5

Designed by Isobel Gillan
Graphics by Ben Cracknell
Illustrations by Kate Simunek

Printed in Great Britain by Martins, the Printers Ltd,
   Berwick upon Tweed
Bound in Great Britain by Hunter and Foulis Ltd, Edinburgh
cover printed in Great Britain by Clays Ltd, St Ives plc

Contents

chapter 1

The Missing Link

I've tried just about every diet there is – the Scarsdale, the Beverly Hills, the F-Plan, the Hip and Thigh – you name it I've tried it. Okay, I might manage to lose some weight. But sooner or later I either get so bored or depressed or just plain ravenous that I slip back into my old ways and that's it – I put it all back on again. Please, please, is there any way out of this vicious circle?

Margaret, aged 31

A familiar story?

Margaret is yet another victim of the infamous 'yo-yo' dieting – the dreaded up and down, up and down, up and down – that plagues so many slimmers.

How often have you been defeated by boredom, misery or insatiable craving – and put all that hard-lost weight back on again?

Over the years, as the resident 'agony doctor' for *Woman* magazine, I've received countless letters like Margaret's, and I've done my best to give helpful advice about sensible healthy low-fat dieting – how to take things slowly and steadily, stay motivated, resist temptation, and find low-calorie snacks and ways of distracting attention from food.

But, somehow, I've always felt that there was something missing – a yawning gap in current slimming recommendations – a crucial missing link.

Then one day, not so long ago, Margaret's letter arrived in my postbag, and, as luck would have it, the very next letter leapt right out at me.

**For two-and-a-half weeks of each month I am a normal
confident woman who finds it easy to stick to a fairly
strict diet in my battle to lose weight.
However, one-and-a-half weeks before my period I
begin to feel fat and ugly, and I eat everything in sight.
Because I believe and think I am ugly and fat, I get
depressed, ratty and very tired. I feel and look bloated
in these days and just cannot stop picking at food –
chocolate, bread, biscuits, etc.
I would very much appreciate your advice on how to
cope with this problem.**

Susan, aged 28

Suddenly, the connection was made in my mind between Susan's and
Margaret's seemingly quite different problems, and I decided there
and then to search the scientific literature for evidence of a possible
link between yo-yo dieting and the menstrual cycle.

The harder I looked the more convinced I became of just how
important the menstrual cycle is to a woman's metabolism, mood,
appetite and weight – whether she's aware of the link or not.

And, most crucially, I found the evidence I was searching for – a
way of harnessing the power of the menstrual cycle to help women
conquer the perennial problem of yo-yo dieting.

This research is the basis of the Body-clock Diet – not just another
slimming diet, but a complete eating and exercise programme tuned
to the subtle changes of your monthly 'biorhythms'. These are the
biochemical ups and downs which are controlled by your body clock.

*Q. Are there certain times of the month when dieting is a real
struggle for you – or goes completely out of the window?*
*Q. Do you ever find yourself craving chocolate, sweet things or
stodge?*
*Q. Are you heartily fed up with your weight constantly yo-yoing
up and down?*
Q. Do you despair at the thought of ever being slim again?

Here, at last, is an eating and exercise programme that not only *understands* why slimming can be so difficult for you – but is also designed to actually make use of your monthly biorhythms to help you lose weight.

Too much to hope for?

Far from it. In the course of my research into this fascinating subject, I asked the readers of *Woman* magazine to write in and tell me about their experiences of food cravings, chocoholism, and dieting problems and the links they have noticed with their menstrual cycle.

I received over 300 replies – many readers giving graphic accounts of the anguish and misery they were suffering. Part of the help and advice they were offered was the opportunity to take part in a trial of one of the Body-clock Diet plans (Plan 1250). The trial diet was compared with a control diet identical in calorie content, menu plans and recipes, but without the crucial link to the menstrual cycle.

Both diets achieved very satisfactory average weight losses as you can see from the chart below – the Body-clock Diet edging just slightly ahead.

But the big difference was that more women preferred the Body-clock Diet and stayed with it longer. Not counting those who had reached their target weight, the 'drop-out' rate for the Body-clock Diet was much lower – only about half that for the control diet. Women particularly liked the Body-clock Diet's adaptability throughout their cycle, the help it gave them in coping with food cravings, and the way in which it seemed much easier to keep to in the week or so before their period.

	Control diet	Body-clock Diet
Average daily calories	1250	1250
Synchronized with periods?	No	Yes
Average monthly weight loss*	4.2 kg (9.2 lb)	4.4 kg (9.8 lb)
Drop-out rate (by 8 weeks)	64%	35%

* This figure is based on dietary adherence up to 8 weeks and includes fluid normally lost in the first 2 weeks of dieting (see page 12)

Although the results were not statistically significant, they were nevertheless most encouraging.

Here's what some of the Body-clock Diet trial slimmers had to say about it:

> **I am going to continue this diet. Hope to lose at least another stone and a half [9.5 kg]. I have now had one period whilst on it and I was amazed at how easy I found it to keep to.**
>
> *Phillippa, aged 37*

> **I was really motivated with the diet and felt much better mentally.**
>
> *Sally, aged 34*

> **Enjoyable and varied and filling, and it's great to be able to have chocolate at the times when I really need it.**
>
> *Michelle, aged 34*

> **The meal plans were really great! Very easy to stick to and filling, and a great choice. The recipes were wonderful, easy to follow and most of them didn't feel like the normal 'Diet' food. Even my husband said it didn't seem as though I was on a diet – which was great!**
>
> *Nina, aged 27*

> **When I had my period I was taken by surprise as I had not had any pre-menstrual symptoms. No tears. No cravings. Just surprise that it was that time already. I definitely put it down to the diet.**
>
> *Wendy, aged 33*

> **I really appreciate being able to eat more to satisfy my cravings in the build-up to my period.**
>
> *Ellen, aged 28*

Will it suit YOU?

The Body-clock Diet is so flexible that it's actually **three slimming plans in one,** to suit as many women as possible.

- 🍎 *Plan 100* – *There's a 'short sharp' version, averaging 1000 calories a day which is best if you have less than a stone to lose*

- 🍎 *Plan 1250* – *a 'moderate pace' version, averaging 1250 calories a day, if you need to lose about 1-3 stones to reach your target .*

- 🍎 *Plan 1500* – *an 'easy does it' version, averaging 1500 calories a day, recommended if you are more than about 3 stones over target, and therefore need to stay on the slimming diet for some months*

Each plan comes complete with set menus and recipes (including vegetarian options), and 'no-fuss' alternatives in case you prefer to concoct your own meals.

What is more, each plan can be adjusted to suit your particular menstrual cycle as closely as possible – whether or not you go the usual 28 days between periods. It can even be made to fit completely irregular periods. And it is especially suitable if you're on the Pill because your cycles should be that much more predictable.

However, as with any other slimming diet, the Body-clock Diet is **NOT** appropriate if:

- 🍎 *you are pregnant, breastfeeding or trying for a baby.*
- 🍎 *you have a severe eating disorder such as anorexia or bulimia.*
- 🍎 *you're under 18.*

In particular, the Body-clock Diet is **NOT** suitable if:

- 🍎 *you are going through, or have been through, the menopause ('change').*
- 🍎 *you are a man!*

But if none of these applies to you, and you want to try the diet that is really challenging the traditional approach to women's slimming, then you need look no further.

How to use this book
In **chapters 1-5**, you can find out why so many other diets fail – and why women are so vulnerable to yo-yo dieting. You will read about the scientific research that has led to the Body-clock Diet and why it is already being talked about as a breakthrough. You will also be able to assess yourself using the 'Know Your Own Body-clock' quiz.

In **chapters 6-10**, you will find the diet itself – with a step-by-step guide on how to follow it, the basic rules, lists of extras and treats, and the three different eating plans, according to your starting weight. You can also savour over fifty delicious recipes.

In **chapters 11 and 12** you can follow the Body-clock Exercise Programme and learn how to use your natural rhythms to maintain your new slimness with the Body-clock StaySlim Plan.

Dig those crazy rhythms
So, don't waste any more time and effort on diets you cannot keep to.

Get in step with the Body-clock Diet, and shake off that surplus weight for good!

chapter 2

Why So Many Diets Fail

Why, oh why?

There are dozens of different diets – if not hundreds – and the chances are you have tried quite a few of them. Why is it then, that despite all the hype and promises, so many of them fail to do the job? Why, even though you have painstakingly counted the calories, weighed the portions, and kept slavishly to the rules, have you still not been able to reach or hold your target weight?

What goes wrong? Is it the diet? Or is it you?

Well, despite what you may or may not think of yourself and your chances of ever being able to lose weight, it's usually the diet that is not right. At least, not right for you.

Let's look into this a bit further...

Crackpot diets

For one thing, there are still quite a few crackpot diets around, based on various unproven theories that frankly do not stand up to serious scientific scrutiny.

Some of them claim that eating particular foods, such as pineapple or grapefruit, will 'cleanse' the system of 'toxins' or 'waste products' that are said to cause the accumulation of that scourge of female hips and thighs, the dimpled disaster 'cellulite'.

Others claim that certain amino acids or enzymes can 'stimulate' the burning of fat.

Still others either recommend particular combinations of nutrients that will somehow block the build-up of fatty tissue, or they warn you against combining other nutrients that will encourage it.

Diets like these may be terribly fashionable and, if they are low enough in calories, you may lose weight very quickly – **but not for long**. They are doomed to ultimate failure, not so much because the science is bogus, but because:

- 🍎 *they are too unnatural and quirky*
  or:
- 🍎 *they are incredibly fiddly*
  or:
- 🍎 *they are grindingly boring*
  or:
- 🍎 *they are all three of these!*

Sooner or later you get fed up with the diet and give it up. In other words, your weight yo-yos back up again.

Frustrating diets

These are the ones which deny you your favourite food. You know the sort of thing. No chocolate. No chips. No cakes or biscuits. No alcohol. Need I go on? Diets this uncompromising usually mean it's yo-yo time again!

Very low calorie diets

These diets are tempting because they can hardly fail to help you lose weight – quite a lot of weight, quite quickly. But after about three weeks things can start to go wrong.

The main problem is that, with **very** low calorie diets, the weight you are losing consists of too much **non-fatty** tissue – like muscle and connective tissue – plus water and essential salts.

This can severely weaken you and be a major shock to the system. Even ordinary everyday exertion can make you feel faint and giddy. This is why doctors recommend that very low calorie diets should not be continued for longer than three or four weeks **at most** and ought to be medically supervised.

Crash diets

Many slimmers try to lose weight fast by eating diets that make all sorts of claims about how many pounds you can shrug off in a week or so.

What they forget to tell you is that the pounds you lose will be nearly all water. Yes, water!

When you first go short of calories – and this applies to all sorts of weight-reducing diets, not just 'crash' diets – your body turns to its emergency supply of instant fuel, a carbohydrate called glycogen stored in your liver. It can convert this very quickly into calories to keep your metabolism (body chemistry) going. Body fat, by contrast, takes much longer to convert into calories.

The trouble is that when glycogen is broken down it releases water, which you then get rid of in your urine. So, you will lose weight, but it will be 'phantom fat', not the real thing.

But wait, it gets worse! As soon as you stop the diet for whatever reason, and start eating normally again, even though you may be being very sensible and careful not to over-indulge, you will suddenly put all those phantom pounds straight back on again! Yes, the dreaded yo-yo! You can't help it. As your liver replenishes its emergency glycogen stores, it takes on water, and on goes the weight.

There are two lessons here. One is that there is no such thing as a crash diet – or even a diet that works any faster than a moderately calorie-reduced diet. You cannot hurry the mobilization of fat – at least not that much. And the second lesson is that when you stop a diet you must expect to gain some of the weight you have lost, and make allowances accordingly.

Plateau-prone diets

The other problem with many slimming diets is that, after about three weeks, you are very likely to hit a 'plateau' – your weight loss levels out and steadfastly refuses to drop any lower.

This is because you have triggered the body's natural self-preservation mechanism for dealing with a shortage of food. Your metabolism has been alerted to the severe lack of calories and has switched into the 'famine response', **slowing itself down** in order to conserve what precious calories it can.

The result is that you burn up fewer and fewer calories, and **store more of them as body fat**. And, just to add insult to injury, if you relax your diet a little and eat more calories, because the famine response still operates for a while, you are much more likely to pile the weight back on again.

As long as you do not go more than about two weeks without some let-up in your diet, even just a brief relaxation of it, you should be able to prevent the dreaded famine response and avoid the otherwise inevitable yo-yo. So the occasional indiscretion or over-indulgence may be no bad thing.

Unrealistic hope diets

Another possible cause of failure – the toughest of all – might be your genes. Recent scientific research has lent support to the theory, propounded by generations of slimmers, that our body shape is at least partly inherited. There seems to be evidence of a 'fatness gene' which programmes our fat cells to maintain a particular degree of plumpness by diverting more of the calories we eat into fatty tissue.

It is as though our bodies have a natural tendency to 'defend' our fatty energy stores. This appears to be a more powerful process in some people than others, and probably more so in women than men.

So, you may be trying to get down to a weight that is simply too low for you – an unrealistic target that is bound to lead to failure. Although standard height-weight charts are a useful guide, your parents' or grandparents' weight at your age might provide a more accurate clue to your own natural target weight.

But don't let this be too easy an excuse! It certainly does not account for all the extra weight you may have put on as a result of years of over-eating or lack of exercise.

Okay-but-not-right-for-you diets

Most of today's slower and more sensible diets are in this category. They are 'slimming plans' which rely on a healthy balance of ordinary foods obtainable from any supermarket or high street, and their calorie content is only moderately reduced – usually by cutting down on fatty or oily things.

You will come across variations of this healthy and sensible approach to slimming in any number of magazines and slimming clubs, and in the many diet booklets issued by the food industry.

These diets are fine as far as they go, and work well for many women, achieving a more-or-less steady weight loss of about 1-2lb a week. **But, unfortunately, they may not work for you.** Why not? Because everybody is different. Not only are you different from other women – but also different in yourself at different times of the day, or the month, or the year. This is true even though you may not realize it. A woman's energies, emotions and metabolism are constantly changing in a rhythmic pattern, particularly every month, whether she's aware of it or not.

This means that, to be most effective for you, a diet has to be geared to all your little ups and downs. Despite any disappointments you may have had with diets in the past, the chances are you are perfectly capable of losing weight, and staying slim, providing you follow a plan that is right for you. A diet that fits you like a glove. A diet that is in step with your rhythms.

The fourth 'M'

Amazingly, none of the world's major diets has so far taken sufficient account of these crucial biorhythms. Although many diet books and slimming club manuals try to get to grips with the three 'Ms' of mood, motivation and metabolism, I couldn't find a single one that is properly tailored to the subtle variations of the fourth 'M' – the menstrual cycle.

The hidden problem

And yet so many women are victims of this scourge. In my survey of the readers of *Woman* magazine, I came across story after story of dedicated and conscientious slimmers being completely thrown off course by the monthly peaks and troughs of their hormones. Here are some typical examples:

I am on a constant diet, but never seem to get anywhere because of this problem. I can control my food intake perfectly well for three weeks, and I manage to shed about 2 lb a week, but in the fourth week I lose control completely and eat every sweet thing in sight – and if it's not in sight I will go out and get it! By the time my period starts and my binge is over, my weight is back to where I started.

Denise, aged 28

Ten days before menstruating I know everything is about to change, especially if I have been trying to diet. I need to eat more, especially between meals. Five days before my period I eat anything in sight. My weight can go up and down half a stone in a month, sometimes more.

Hilary, no age given

I am about a stone and a half overweight. For the first three weeks after my period I have my eating under control, and then just before my period I have to eat everything – chocolate, cake, biscuits, jam sandwiches. My oldest boy is just beginning to twig that it's me who's eating his jelly babies!

Susan, aged 27

About a week before my period I feel so fed up and irritable that I just think 'What the heck!' and stuff myself like a pig.

Sarah, aged 32

The only time since puberty that I can remember having any control and eating normally for more than two weeks at a stretch was when I was pregnant with each of my two children.

Maggie, no age given

From the day my period starts and for the following two weeks I can diet successfully, and normally lose 7-10lb. But for the two weeks leading up to my period I stuff my face and end up putting all the weight back on. Chocolate is what I crave most, and it isn't unusual for me to make my long-suffering husband drive to a garage at midnight to get me some!

Daniele, aged 29

Rhythms and blues

But why are your mood, motivation, metabolism and menstrual cycle all so closely linked? And what can be done to break the vicious circle?

In the past few years startling new evidence has emerged which begins to make sense of the whole conundrum. It comes from research into the anthropology, psychology and biochemistry of the four 'Ms'.

It also comes from the relatively new science of chronobiology – the study of body-clocks and biorhythms – which has begun to reveal the profound effects of day and night, winter and summer, and, most important of all, the fourth 'M' – the menstrual cycle.

In the next two chapters I shall try to explain how this complicated jigsaw fits together, and also how dieting for women can never be quite the same again.

So, read on to discover...

- *how premenstrual food cravings are normal and natural*
- *how chocolate and sweet things can prevent bingeing*
- *how monthly ups and downs can be harnessed to prevent yo-yo dieting.*

chapter 3

Body-clock Blues

What exactly is your body-clock?
How does it control your biorhythms and mood?
And what effect can it have on your cravings and weight?

In this chapter and the next we shall be looking at some of the scientific background to the Body-clock Diet. Not in great detail – but enough to see why daily, seasonal and especially monthly biorhythms are now being recognised as such an important factor in dieting for women.

However, if you'd rather skip the science, and get straight down to the practicalities, I suggest you turn to the self-assessment quiz in Chapter 5 – Know Your Own Body-clock.

What is your body-clock?

Scientists have been looking for some sort of timing mechanism in the brains of humans and animals for over a hundred years. There are so many bodily changes that happen in a rhythmic way throughout the day, month and year that there surely has to be a central control – like the conductor of a vast orchestra keeping the beat.

But it's only in the past decade, with improving technology, that the search has really begun to pinpoint the body-clock in the base of the brain. We now know that it's situated in an area called the hypothalamus, right alongside the appetite centre and sleep centre, and just above the pituitary gland which controls so many basic functions, including the menstrual cycle.

The body-clock is actually a network of special cells which, in a way still not fully understood, releases chemical messengers, rhythmically rising and falling with the passage of time – in effect the 'ticking' of the clock. These messengers act as signals to the other centres in the hypothalamus and the pituitary gland, to switch dozens of bodily processes on and off at the right times. In other words, your body-clock 'conducts' your biorhythms.

...and what exactly are biorhythms?

The word 'biorhythms' is simply the scientific shorthand for biological rhythms, a general term for the many thousands of regular fluctuations that occur in the natural world of plants and animals. But as far as we humans are concerned, biorhythms are the regular ups and downs of our body chemistry which shape our lives each day, month and year.

We shall be looking more closely at the typical female pattern of biorhythms in a moment. But first, let me clear up a possible source of confusion. The term 'biorhythms' first hit the public in a big way in the 1970s when it was used by the followers of a now discredited theory to describe physical, emotional and intellectual cycles of exactly twenty-three, twenty-eight and thirty-three days respectively. At that time, these so-called 'biorhythms' were a great fad and enthusiasts took great pains to plan their lives according to their 'biorhythm predictions' calculated from the precise date and time of their birth.

However, although there was an element of truth in the idea of fluctuating mind and body rhythms, such precise and rigid calculations were soon shown to be completely false. People's minds and bodies simply don't work in such a predictable way. Yes, we all have a body-clock – but it's far from being a highly accurate chronometer. In fact, it gains and loses like crazy and can be knocked out of kilter by all sorts of things, from the common cold to a night of revelry, and from jet-lag to a broken love affair.

Everyone's different

Your body-clock and the biorhythms it conducts are crucial in shaping your life and, as we shall see, they're particularly crucial in shaping your body. But no two people are exactly the same in the way their body-clock works. Nor is each person's body-clock entirely regular.

Nevertheless, the growing science of chronobiology – the study of biorhythms – has revealed rhythmic patterns which are typical for the average woman.

As far as your mood, appetite and weight are concerned, the most important rhythm is almost certainly your monthly cycle. But first let's look at the influence of your daily and seasonal rhythms.

Your daily rhythms

Here are the most typical rhythms throughout the twenty-four hours for the average woman. In fact, most people's daily body-clock tends to run slightly slow, and lags a little behind each day. But fortunately the bedside alarm clock, the amount of daylight, and other daily pressures force us to keep up to speed.

- *alertness:* 'larks' are more alert in the early morning and early evening: 'owls' around midday and late evening.
- *mood:* usually lowest in mid-afternoon and late evening.
- *appetite:* most at midday and early evening.
- *food craving:* peaks in mid-afternoon and late evening.
- *blood sugar:* peaks about 30 minutes after sugary food and 1-2 hours after starchy or fatty foods. Low blood sugar is most likely to occur 45-60 minutes after something sugary.
- *metabolism:* higher in the afternoon than the morning, decreasing during the evening and night.
- *temperature:* lowest in the small hours, increases throughout the day and is highest mid-evening, but by no more than 0.5°C (1°F).
- *heart-rate:* fastest mid-morning and early evening; slowest in mid-afternoon and at night.
- *blood pressure:* highest in the late morning; lowest in the small hours.
- *fluid retention:* increases slightly throughout the day; and decreases during the night.
- *weight:* goes up and down by a few pounds during the 24 hours. The average for women is 900 g (2 lb), but it can be 3 kg (7 lb) or more.

Your 24-Hour Symphony

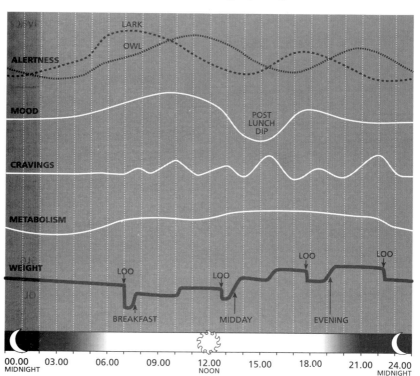

How do daily rhythms affect dieting?

Not an easy question to answer. During the average 24 hours, there is so much rising and falling and pushing and pulling and to-ing and fro-ing of the various bodily functions, that it has been an incredibly difficult conundrum for the scientists to sort out. What is more, everybody is different, and these rhythms will vary to some extent from person to person.

Nevertheless, what does seem clear is that the all-too-familiar 'weak' times as far as slimming is concerned – the times when you are most likely to crave or binge – usually coincide with your mood slumps – for most women mid-afternoon and late evening. So, no surprises there.

Research by Dr Judith Wurtman of the Massachusetts Institute of Technology in the USA has clearly demonstrated that the mid-afternoon slump (also known as the 'post-lunch dip') can be eliminated or helped by having a high-starch midday meal – a chunky sandwich, jacket potato, rice or pasta dish for instance. This effect seems to be enhanced if you keep the protein content of the meal to a minimum (it is thought to compete with the mood-lifting effect of starch). Similarly, the bedtime craving can be eased with a late evening starchy snack, such as your favourite (non-sugary!) cereal.

You can also see how much your weight may fluctuate throughout the 24 hours – which is why, whenever you weigh yourself (no more than once a week!), you should always do so at the same time of day.

Your Seasonal Rhythm

Another, less well known, job for your body-clock is to control the changes that affect your mind and body throughout the year.

These annual rhythms are nowhere near as important to humans as they are to other mammals, particularly those living in the parts of the world where there are very distinct seasons. This is because the seasons dictate their breeding cycle, and everything has to be timed so that the young are born at the best time of the year for their survival – usually spring or summer.

In cold climates, there is also a pressing need for most mammals to stoke up on food and fatten themselves up in the autumn as a source of energy to last them through the winter. And, of course, many smaller mammals save energy by hibernating – they curl up in a ball and go to sleep until spring.

The same need to link in with the seasons no longer applies to humans – although it probably did in prehistoric days. We don't, for instance, have such clear-cut annual breeding rhythms – thank goodness. Can you imagine what life would be like if all babies were born in the spring? Just think of the queue at the antenatal clinic!

But there is some evidence that we still retain a vestige of the annual rhythm for eating high energy foods and hibernating.

Humans hibernating?

That's right. Many women notice a distinct difference in their usual energy level, mood, appetite, and weight between summer and winter.

- *Do you feel more tired and listless in the winter months?*
- *Do you tend to sleep and eat more at that time of year?*
- *Do you usually put on more weight in winter?*

If you answer yes to any of these, and most women do, you are almost certainly being influenced by the biochemical changes of your seasonal rhythm. In its mildest form, you may simply be a 'winter weighty', putting on 3 kg (7 lb) or more through lack of exercise and too much high-calorie food in the winter months. But if the symptoms are quite troublesome, you may be a victim of SAD – seasonal affective disorder or 'winter blues' – the human equivalent of hibernation.

The winter of your discontent?

SAD is a form of low spirits that can range from being a very mild lethargy to quite deep depression – and it is four times more common in women than men.

In winter, SAD sufferers feel weary and dreary. They lack energy, can't 'get going', their concentration wavers, they find it harder to enjoy themselves. By late winter or early spring they feel really low.

The one thing that gives them some comfort, at least for a short while, is food – particularly high carbohydrate, sugary and starchy things. A classic problem for anyone with even just a hint of winter blues is a real craving for sweets, chocolates, cakes and biscuits. If you have premenstrual carbohydrate cravings, the chances are they are noticeably worse in winter.

So, what's the answer then?

This is where the Body-clock Diet comes in. The eating plans are specially designed to help you cope with the cravings, and you will find a range of choices to suit the season. Also, the Body-clock Exercise Programme has been designed to be flexible enough to keep you active whatever the weather.

Your Monthly Rhythm

Now we come to the big one as far as mood, food and your body-clock is concerned – your monthly rhythm, the menstrual cycle. Whether or not your periods are regular, whether or not you are on the Pill, your monthly rhythm has more of an effect on your emotions, appetite and metabolism than perhaps you realize.

Of course, many women are hardly aware of the physical and mental changes that take place throughout the month, apart from the period itself, and may not be in the least bothered by them. But, for others, the monthly cycle can be a dominating influence in their lives – not least by making all the difference between success or failure in dieting.

A taboo subject

And yet there seems to be a deafening silence surrounding the subject of periods and weight control. It is all too rarely mentioned in diet books or at slimming clubs – almost as if it is somehow 'politically incorrect'. Nevertheless, the power of periods can't be denied. Let's look more closely at what is happening inside a woman's body and mind throughout the month.

Basics of the menstrual cycle

By about the age of eighteen, most women have settled down to a fairly regular pattern of periods which continues, apart from interruptions with pregnancies, until the approach of the menopause ('change of life') at around fifty.

The usual length of the complete menstrual cycle, from one period to the next, can vary from about twenty-one to about thirty-five days – but more women have a cycle of about twenty-eight days than any other duration.

Even though you may usually be quite regular, your period might quite often be a day or two later or earlier if you are excessively tired, worried, stressed, ill or jet-lagged.

For as many as one in four women, the periods are not at all regular, but are variable and unpredictable, especially for the first few years after starting menstruation and for a year or so before the menopause. They may be light one month and heavy, perhaps with flooding, the next.

A typical cycle

Here are the main events of a typical 28-day cycle:

Menstruation – about four days. Day One of the cycle is taken as the first day of bleeding. The duration of the period itself, the cramps and bleeding, can vary from one to ten days but the average is four. The 'blood' is actually the disintegrating spongy lining of the womb.

Phase A – lasting about 14 days. Beginning on Day One or soon after (and including the period). Proper name, the follicular phase – so-called because about twenty follicles (egg-containing cysts) on the surface of each of the two ovaries are 'ripened' by the action of a hormone from the pituitary gland at the base of the brain. These ripening follicles produce more and more oestrogen, which stimulates the womb to grow a new lining. One of the follicles becomes larger and more mature than all the others, like a bubble on the ovary.

Ovulation (egg release). About fourteen days before the next period is due, another hormone from the pituitary gland switches off the oestrogen, and 'bursts' the mature follicle, releasing its egg into the fallopian tube, where it is wafted towards the womb.

Phase B – lasing about 7-10 days. Proper name, the luteal phase. Starts after ovulation. The empty follicle becomes a gland *(corpus luteum)* secreting oestrogen and, more importantly, progesterone, the 'pregnancy hormone' which prepares the lining of the womb to receive the egg if it is fertilized. But if fertilization doesn't take place, or the fertilized egg fails to implant in the womb, the luteal phase gives way to Phase C...

Phase C – lasting about 4-7 days, or more. This is the premenstrual phase, usually starting on about Day 21 to 24. The levels of oestrogen and progesterone suddenly plummet to very low levels, usually causing mood changes and other symptoms (see overleaf) and eventually triggering the period – 'the bloody tears of a disappointed womb'.

Changes in the Body during the Menstrual Cycle

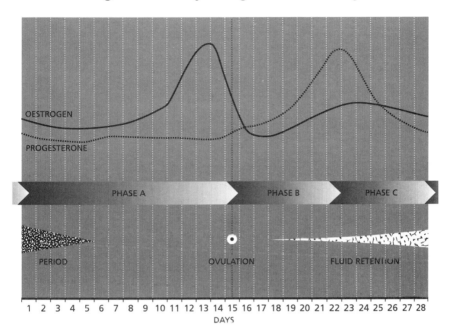

So, for a typical 28-day cycle, each week follows roughly this pattern:

Week 1: Period
Phase A begins
Week 2: Phase A continues
Week 3: Ovulation
Phase B begins
Week 4: Phase C begins

However, if your cycle is nearer five weeks long, you would usually have a longer Phase A – perhaps lasting up to about 21days. And if your cycle is only three weeks long, you may spend little over a week in Phase A.

Other changes

A number of other physical and psychological changes occur at various phases of the menstrual cycle, some of which may have an effect on how you manage to stick to your diet.

Mood. Most women feel a little edgy and less cheerful in the days before their period. Some become quite anxious, tearful, irritable or depressed (see Premenstrual Syndrome on page 28).

Phase C is also the time when many women feel less energetic, have difficulty concentrating, and may notice that their ability to co-ordinate complicated movements is not as good as usual. Women often have a rather negative opinion of themselves at this time, and feel frumpy and unattractive.

Appetite. Scientists at the University of Toronto have surveyed a random sample of women aged eighteen to forty-one and found that both food intake and body weight are significantly higher during Phases B and C than during Phase A.

Food cravings. Over 90 per cent of women have food cravings from time to time, usually fancying something chocolatey, sweet, or stodgy. In most cases the cravings are strongest in the second half of the menstrual cycle, with a peak time of four or five days before each period. Researchers at the University of Maryland, USA, have shown that this is also the favourite time for salty foods.

Metabolism. Although a woman's daytime resting metabolic rate does not change much throughout her cycle, Dutch scientists have found that at night it is increased in the ten nights before each period, by up to 10 per cent. This means your body burns off calories more efficiently in the second half of your cycle than the first half.

Temperature. Linked to this increase in metabolic rate, your temperature rises by about 1 degree C in the second half of your cycle. Scientists at Glasgow Royal Infirmary in Scotland persuaded twenty-five women to wear special 'thermometric' bras and measured their breast temperature throughout the month. There was a definite but gradual rise in temperature after ovulation (about Day 15), and a quite sudden drop at the onset of their period. This temperature rise tends to be a little higher for women with PMS .

Skin and hair. The skin and scalp become greasier, and the hair lanker, in the latter part of the cycle.

Physical energy. Most women feel much less inclined to take exercise in the second half of their cycle than in the first. Enthusiasm, energy, endurance and co-ordination all tend to be reduced at that time of the month. The best time for physical activity is likely to be immediately after each period.

These are usually the most noticeable changes, but you may be aware of others. A good idea is to make a note of them in your diary – or use the chart below. You can refer to this later when you are choosing meal plans and snacks to avoid cravings.

Your Personal Pattern

Use this chart to plot the main changes that you experience throughout each month.

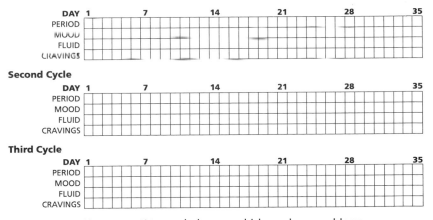

Use a cross ✗ to mark days on which you have problems,
counting the first day of your period as Day 1.

Premenstrual syndrome (PMS)

It is perfectly normal for you to experience some premenstrual disturbances of mind or body. About 95 per cent of women are aware of various changes in themselves in the second half of their cycle, especially in the few days before their period.

These changes may amount to very little, and cause no trouble whatsoever. Or they may be completely disruptive, and make life a misery for the woman and those around her. But, more often than not, they will be somewhere in between these two extremes, giving rise to a variety of symptoms, some more bothersome than others.

Here is a list of typical premenstrual symptoms:

- *mood swings*
- *food cravings*
- *breast swelling and tenderness*
- *a bloated abdomen*
- *puffy face and hands*
- *tension headaches*
- *migraine*
- *irritable bowel syndrome*
- *fainting*
- *fatigue*
- *visual blurring*
- *thirst*
- *urinary urgency*

Any combination of these is usually referred to as the premenstrual syndrome (PMS) – although the mood swings may be called premenstrual 'tension'.

Why some women suffer from PMS and others do not is something of a mystery. It seems to be linked to an imbalance of oestrogen and yet another hormone, androgen, the so-called 'male' hormone that all women have a little of in their system. For some reason the androgen gets the upper hand in the latter part of the cycle. PMS is more likely to affect women in their thirties and forties, perhaps because their oestrogen is beginning to fade a little.

Let us look at some of these PMS symptoms in more detail:

Fluid retention. Virtually all women have some fluid retention in the days before their period. It usually takes the form of slight puffiness of the face, hands, breasts, abdomen and legs, and tends to increase during the day, easing off again during the night.

The average woman gains and loses about 1-1.5 kg (2-3 lb) of fluid over each twenty-four hours during the last week of her cycle, but in severe cases this premenstrual daily yo-yo can be anything up to about 6.5.kg (14 lb). Your waist measurement can increase by anything from 2.5 to 15 cm (1 to 6 inches).

Not surprisingly, women with marked fluid retention feel 'bloated' and 'puffy', and have to take off their rings and wear looser clothes. But many of the other typical symptoms of PMS are thought to be due, at least partly, to excess fluid in various organs, including the brain and bowels.

Fluid retention is caused by the high levels of progesterone and oestrogen in the last week or two of the cycle, but there is an added factor which might make you even more susceptible. Many experts believe that being more than about 9 kg (20 lb) overweight puts pressure on the veins, and fools the fluid-control system into retaining even more fluid.

This would mean that the more overweight you are, the more fluid retention you are likely to suffer – and, conversely, the more excess weight you can shed, the less you will be bothered by puffy tissues and feeling bloated.

Mood changes. Up to nine out of ten women have some monthly mood changes. The usual tendency is to become more tense, irritable, tetchy, snappy, tearful and depressed in the days before each period. One woman in three is driven to seek medical help for these and other premenstrual symptoms, and one woman in twenty is so incapacitated that she has to take time off work.

Listen to this typical example from a mother of three:

> **I am unfortunately a sufferer of mood swings, especially the four days before a period. I am okay one minute, then really nasty and hateful the next. .... My children are frightened to speak to me, as is my husband. They can all tell when it's the dreaded 'monthlies'.**
>
> *Jo, aged 27*

Some women talk about their 'Jekyll and Hyde' character – or even feeling 'murderous'.

> **The worst thing is my mood swings. What I would normally consider the most insignificant of problems seems during this time to become quite big and upsetting. I feel sudden bursts of hate towards anyone who gets in my way in shops and traffic. I feel as if I could quite easily punch someone in the face. I feel I want to be alone, and yet I feel so lonely I keep bursting into tears.**
>
> *Angela, aged 37*

Food cravings. These are very much linked to low moods, and usually take the form of an intense desire to eat sugary, stodgy or fatty things. Chocolate is the runaway favourite. Satisfying the craving seems to have a definite, if only temporary, cheering or soothing effect. We shall explore this crucial link between mood and food more deeply in the next chapter.

Breast changes. Most women experience some 'fullness' and perhaps tenderness in their breasts in the second half of their cycle. Many say that their breasts feel uncomfortably 'heavy' or 'tight'. They may also notice a general lumpiness. The swelling may be enough to need the next bra size. Some of this increase is due to swollen milk glands, but most is fluid retention.

Headaches. These are usually 'tension headaches' or migraine attacks, and can be pretty crippling.

Relief for PMS
Apart from losing weight and staying slim, what other ways are there of helping to relieve the symptoms of PMS? Well, despite the fact that this distressing condition has been plaguing womankind since long before there were any doctors, I am afraid that medical science has still to discover a safe and satisfactory remedy for it. And, as is usual

when there is no sure-fire cure for an ailment, a whole range of self-help treatments and complementary therapies have been advocated.

Some of these do help some sufferers some of the time – and for that reason are worth trying. But be prepared to be disappointed.

A high carbohydrate diet. Lots of sweet, sugary or starchy things. More carbohydrate and less protein certainly seem to help women who have mood swings and cravings. The trick is to make these changes without wrecking your diet.

Frequent but smaller meals. These help to prevent low blood sugar, mood swings and hunger.

Cut down on salt? This is often recommended, even by doctors, and yet the evidence is not at all clear-cut. Some experts say that less sodium (a key component of salt) in the week before your period will help to reduce fluid retention, because body water and sodium tend to go hand in hand.

But there is no convincing evidence that PMS sufferers have excess sodium in their system. Indeed some doctors have argued that more sodium may be needed premenstrually, not less, because the excess fluid has to be accompanied by sodium, and if there is not enough to go round it will be taken from vital processes, making you dizzy and headachy. My advice is to try both approaches to see if either of them works for you.

Regular Exercise. Canadian research has shown that regular exercise throughout the whole cycle really can help PMS symptons: it enhances concentration, improves negative moods and prevents food cravings. It can even reduce the pain of the period itself. It doesn't have to be particularly vigorous – gentle, moderate, rhythmic activity like walking, cycling or swimming is best for most women. However, if bad temper and severe tension are the main problems, it's worth trying hard aerobics or some other more vigorous exercise.

Unfortunately, the premenstrual phase is the very time when you probably feel least like exerting yourself. Studies on women athletes have shown that their co-ordination and endurance are significantly impaired during those premenstrual days.

But, having said that, if you are a PMS sufferer, the only prize you are out to win is to lose weight and feel better. So, it is well worth making the effort to get moving. Follow the Body-clock Exercise Programme in Chapter 11.

Evening primrose oil. This nutritional supplement is widely advocated as helpful for PMS. The active ingredient is gamma-linolenic acid (GLA). Another even richer source of GLA is the oil from starflower seeds.

Evidence for the benefits of evening primrose oil is mixed. Most studies agree that it helps premenstrual breast tenderness. But there is less agreement on its usefulness for the many other symptoms of PMS. It seems to help some women, but not others.

Nevertheless, just because its value has not been clearly proven does not mean it would not work for you – so the best thing is to try it for yourself. Capsules of evening primrose oil are widely available from chemists and health food shops, but are not cheap. Some doctors recommend that it is taken together with vitamin B6.

Vitamin B6. Also called pyridoxine, one of the B family of vitamins, and widely advocated as a remedy for PMS. It plays a part in many vital functions, including the metabolism of essential amino acids and fatty acids. It is thought to help many PMS symptoms, especially the depression, poor concentration and headaches, but, as with evening primrose oil, the evidence is controversial. It probably helps some women to a limited extent if taken for at least three days before the start of each period and for two days after.

The vitamin is fairly plentiful in a normal healthy diet, and few people are short of it. Rich sources are: red meat, liver, kidney, fish, avocados, bananas, dried fruit, yeast extract. It is also obtainable in tablet form from chemists, usually in combination with other vitamins, but care should be taken not to exceed the recommended dose.

Magnesium. The level of this mineral has been found to be low in women with PMS and this deficiency is thought to interfere with the metabolism of certain essential fatty acids. It may also affect blood sugar levels. A magnesium supplement, in the form of tablets or capsules, may help some sufferers, particularly if taken with evening primrose oil and vitamin B6 – but once again the evidence is not very strong.

Other nutritional supplements. The most frequently advocated are vitamin E, zinc and selenium. The evidence for these is even less impressive than for the supplements I have already mentioned. But again they may be worth trying in moderate doses.

What about diuretics? Although diuretic medication (to increase urine output) will undoubtedly remove excess fluid from your body, it does not usually help the fluid retention of PMS. This is because it takes fluid from the bloodstream rather than the tissues, and simply makes you very thirsty.

So, my view is that diuretics are best avoided. Not only are there possible side-effects, but there is also a risk of 'rebound' fluid retention when you stop the medication.

...and the Pill? If you are on the Pill you may have noticed that your premenstrual mood tends to be rather lower than it was before, or that you stay down for a bit longer. This is a common problem with the Pill, although it varies from woman to woman and Pill to Pill.

The mood-lowering effect is probably the result of fluid retention caused by oestrogen in the Pill. A similar but rather milder effect can happen with HRT (hormone replacement therapy).

The mood and food conspiracy. So your biorhythms, whether daily, monthly or annual, can have a profound effect on your well-being and your weight. With all three rhythms, one of the most crucial factors is your mood. In the next chapter, we explore the reasons why mood and food are so intimately connected, and why they can so easily conspire against you.

chapter 4

Mood and Food

Biorhythms are very much a fact of life – especially for women. They orchestrate the ebb and flow of your hormones and brain chemicals. They govern your energy, appetite and mood. They lift you up and they drag you down. And they are crucial in your battle to get slim and stay slim.

In this chapter we will see how these factors interact with each other, and why your mood is so important in dictating your eating habits. We will look at the latest scientific evidence which explains:

- *why particular foods are such a comfort*
- *why food cravings are not a weakness, but a strength*
- *how the Body-clock works with your food cravings, not against them.*

But first of all let us look a little more closely at what is happening in your head, and why your mood and food seem so often to conspire against you.

Comfort eating

Most people are familiar enough with the idea of 'comfort foods'. Foods which help us feel better when we are down, upset or in pain. Foods which cheer us up. Foods which calm us down. Foods which help us feel that life may not be too bad after all.

Sweet things in particular have earned themselves a place as great comforters, from that first jelly baby when we fell and grazed our knee to the consolation box of chocs when we failed our driving test or muffed an exam.

Dr Larry Christensen, a psychologist at Texas A&M University, has studied the comfort foods chosen by people with various types of low mood. His research shows that sufferers most often use simple carbohydrates (sugary things) to help lift their spirits, and that these seem to work, at least for a while. This 'feelgood' effect of sugary things can quickly sow the seeds of sweetness craving.

Scientists at McMaster University, Ontario, have investigated over a thousand younger adults of both sexes, and have made the following important discoveries:

- *an incredible 97 per cent of younger women admit to food cravings.*
- *one-third of women link their cravings directly to their menstrual cycle.*

The same study has also clearly demonstrated that chocolate is far and away the most frequently craved food, especially by women. Next in popularity come other sweet things. Surprisingly, dieting does not appear to make the cravings any worse.

Yet another study, this time by researchers at the University of Pennsylvania, has found that:

- *about 50 per cent of younger women crave chocolate, and, of these, about 50 per cent crave it most intensely in the week before their period.*

Of course, chocolate and other sweet things are not every woman's favourite. Other things can be yearned for instead. Stodgy, starchy things that are satisfyingly filling, perhaps, like a chunky sandwich or a bowlful of cereal or pasta. Or fatty, like a fry-up. Or meaty, like a good hefty steak. Or milky, like a bedtime drink. In the second half of their cycle, women often crave something salty, like crisps or salted peanuts.

But survey after survey shows that for most women the classic comforter is something sweet or starchy, or both. Let's find out why.

Sweet talk

Biologists believe that humans have a naturally sweet tooth because we evolved as hunter-gatherers and our diet was largely vegetarian – roots, shoots and fruits – with only an occasional piece of meat if the spear-party struck lucky. Sweet succulent things were much sought after, and provided extra calories – vital when food was scarce.

Therefore, the biologists say, we instinctively revert to sweet things in times of crisis. It's a fundamental drive – a survival mechanism – and, although people without a sweet tooth have managed to suppress this instinct, it's still there lurking beneath the surface.

What is more, claim the biologists, the reason why sweetness craving is much stronger for women than for men is linked to their function as potential mothers. Ovulation only happens if there is enough fuel in the form of glycogen (stored carbohydrate) and bodyfat to sustain the energy demands of pregnancy. Therefore it is biologically advantageous for women to be well-fed and plump.

This could also explain the sweetness cravings in the second half of the monthly cycle – the time when progesterone is preparing the body for pregnancy. Any newly fertilized egg would need a well-nourished mother to increase its chances of successful implantation and survival in the womb.

Certainly women are naturally plumper than men, and the fat stores in the breasts, hips and thighs are hormonally controlled to hold on to their fat as tenaciously as possible in times of starvation. The biologists call the fat in these places 'defended' fat – the body does its best to defend all attempts to dislodge it. As any female slimmer knows, these are the hardest places to lose fat from, and the first places to put it back on again when you stop dieting.

In prehistoric times, when survival was a more pressing problem than slimming, the quickest way of replenishing these defended fat stores would have been to eat some sugary food. So, the biologists have given you a wonderful excuse. Your liking for sweet things is a basic instinct programmed into your genes, and is a very natural and very female feature.

Just think – no more guilt!

All in the mind?

An alternative explanation for sugar-craving comes from the psychologists. It all goes back to early childhood, they say (they would, wouldn't they?).

For instance, every time you cried with hunger as a baby, and were rewarded with warm milk, you developed a deep-seated fondness for things sweet. Why sweet? Because, human milk contains more lactose (milk sugar) than that of most other mammals, and its predominant taste is sweet. The same applies to formula feeds, adapted to mimic human milk. It is here, at the breast or bottle, that comfort eating begins.

Indeed, some psychologists have gone further and argued that, because these milk feeds are a combination of sugar and fat, comfort foods later in life are also likely to be combinations of sugar and fat – biscuits or buttered toast and jam for example, and of course the ultimate comforter – chocolate.

But it is as older babies and toddlers that we really get hooked on sweetness. Sweets, sugary snacks and sweet drinks given as a comfort, pacifier or reward have a powerful effect on the psyche, plugging the taste of sweetness straight into our subconscious mind, a 'direct line' with our emotions. Even those people who do not have much of a sweet tooth still retain this basic link, say the psychologists, although they have learnt to suppress it and 're-train' their taste buds to manage with much less sugar.

Dr Andrew Hill, a psychologist at Leeds University, England, has shown that food craving is more likely to be triggered by a low mood than by hunger or dieting. Boredom, irritability or anxiety are the negative emotions that really get cravers craving.

This is certainly borne out by many of the letters I received in my survey. Here is one example:

> **I crave the chocolate because I am so fed up and disillusioned with life, and chocolate makes me feel better. I feel so guilty afterwards, but it doesn't stop me. I have a debate in my head about whether to eat the chocolate or not, and the chocolate always wins.**
>
> *Maureen, aged 32*

The biochemical discoveries

The biologists and psychologists have provided us with plausible explanations which are no doubt part of the true picture. But it is recent discoveries by the biochemists and neurophysiologists that are really shedding light not only on sugar-craving but the whole mood-food connection.

Over the past few years, these scientists have begun to discover much more about the biochemistry of the human brain. In particular, they have looked at some of our most fundamental emotions and drives – happiness, sadness, hunger, desire and energy – and have charted the effects of different types of food on various chemical substances in the brain that seem to play a crucial part in the way we feel these things.

Sugar perks

Take sugar for example. Biochemists see sweet things as providing 'instant energy'. The various types of sugar in our food are 'simple' carbohydrates which are rapidly broken down and absorbed into our bloodstream, giving our brains a welcome 'hit' of energy when our blood glucose level has been bumping along the bottom of its normal range. In this way, they say, sugary things can perk us up – at least for a while.

And not just sugary things. Complex carbohydrates too – starchy things such as bread, biscuits, cakes, potatoes, pasta and rice. These can have a similar but slightly delayed effect. Starch consists of strings of glucose-like sugar-units disguised in a fluffy, powdery, non-sweet form, and it does not take your digestive enzymes very long to release and absorb this hidden sugar. You can test this for yourself by putting a little cornflour on your tongue – within a moment or two the enzyme amylase in your saliva starts to break down the starch in the cornflour into glucose with its distinctive sweet taste.

In the early 1980s, researchers at Massachusetts Institute of Technology decided to investigate the links between food and mood. One of the first things they discovered was that sugary or starchy foods stimulate the brain to release a 'neurotransmitter' or chemical messenger called serotonin (seer-o-toe-nin) which acts as a natural built-in tranquillizer. It helps to calm and soothe the troubled mind. It also reduces the craving for sugary and starchy foods.

The serotonin connection

Serotonin acts as a mood-food regulator. When the level of serotonin in the brain falls too low it creates a feeling of anxiety, irritability and restlessness. A low level of serotonin also switches on the drive to eat sugary or starchy things. Once eaten and absorbed into the system, these then increase the level of serotonin, and the craving subsides.

So serotonin seems to be the key link between mood and food, at least as far as sugary and starchy things are concerned. Through the serotonin connection a low mood can cause carbohydrate cravings – and satisfying those cravings can restore some degree of serenity. Unfortunately, with sugary things, that may be for only a very short while.

Serotonin Levels and your Mood

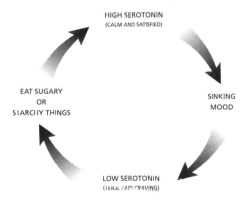

HIGH SEROTONIN
(CALM AND SATISFIED)

SINKING
MOOD

EAT SUGARY
OR
STARCHY THINGS

LOW SEROTONIN
(TENSE AND CRAVING)

Sugar – the false friend

The trouble is that, okay, sweet things definitely perk me up. But an hour later I feel dreadful again. No, I actually feel worse than before. Hungrier and much more ratty and miserable.

Anne, aged 31

Does that sound familiar to you? Do you find sugar to be a false friend? Do sugary things only lift you for a short time before dropping you like a stone? Do you keep needing sugary snacks all day long to fend off the plunging lows that sugar can cause?

The 'sugar dumps'. The problem here is the famous 'sugar dumps', or what doctors refer to as 'reactive hypoglycaemia' – a sudden low blood sugar level caused, paradoxically, by eating too much sugar on an empty stomach. It happens like this.

If you are hungry because you have not eaten for some time, a sugary snack – like a chocolate bar – will push your blood sugar level way up high. This makes your pancreas panic and release lots of insulin in an effort to keep your blood sugar under control. The result is your blood sugar slumps and you feel hungry and miserable. So you are tempted to have another chocolate bar, and the whole vicious cycle repeats itself.

How to avoid the 'sugar dumps'. There are basically three ways of doing this.

One is to avoid sugary things – not easy if the cravings become really intense.

Another way is not to go too long without food. Reactive hypoglycaemia is much more likely if sugar is eaten on an empty stomach. So it is important not to miss meals. You must have at least three meals a day, and at times of intense cravings, especially in your premenstrual phase, it is best to have three snack meals in between. The Body-clock Diet provides these.

The Sugar Dumps

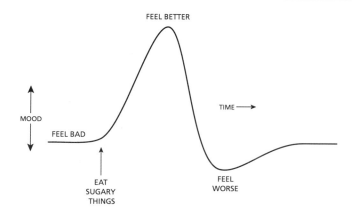

The third way is to eat a starchy food either instead of, or along with, the sugary food. As we have seen, starchy foods have a similar serotonin-boosting and uplifting effect to sugar. But because the starch takes longer to digest and is usually wrapped in fibre it has a delayed action or 'time release' effect. Unlike sugar, it does not trigger the pancreas panic pumping of insulin, and avoids the ghastly fall of blood sugar.

> Dr Judith Wurtman, a research nutritionist at the Massachusetts Institute of Technology, has found that a high carbohydrate starchy meal starts to improve depression, tension, anger, confusion, sadness, fatigue and irritability within thirty minutes of eating. The effect is sustained for up to two hours. She has also found that a lunch of mainly starchy carbohydrate helps to prevent the 'post-lunch dip'.

Why is chocolate so addictive?
A good question. Apart from the sugar, what is so special about chocolate? Why are so many women driven to become such desperate chocoholics – especially just before their period?

It starts about twelve days before my period. I have to have it. I will have had a bath and be ready for bed and will have tried to get the better of myself, but it's no use, on goes my coat over my nightdress, and out I dash for my quick fix of choc from the late-night shop.

Diane, no age given

Before my period I have an insatiable desire for chocolate (not sweet things, it has to be chocolate). I've tried those low-calorie bars, but they don't have the same taste. After two or three bars of the real thing I feel so relaxed and calm – it must be something in the chocolate itself.

Jane, aged 27

And Lisa, aged 31, is badly hooked too:

> **My diet goes completely out of the window during the four days before my period. I can eat five bars of chocolate at any one time and still crave for more. It's an obsession that completely takes me over. I've tried having diet hot chocolate drinks – but they don't help. I've tried having a biscuit every four hours, but that didn't help either. Nothing gets rid of the constant nagging for chocolate, apart from chocolate – real chocolate. My husband keeps finding multi-pack bars of chocolate that I've hidden in odd places all around the house, so that I'm never too far from a fix.**

Is there a magic ingredient? Perhaps, but nothing has been scientifically demonstrated so far, apart from the serotonin-boosting effect of sugar. Some experts believe that the fat in chocolate can increase the brain's endorphin level – another 'feelgood' hormone – but why then don't other fatty foods have the same effect?

Chocolate does contain mild stimulants in the form of theobromine and caffeine – but much less than in tea or coffee, neither of which have the 'addictive' powers of chocolate. And it also contains phenylethylamine – but the effects of this on the brain are not clear.

So, quite why chocolate is so seductive is truly a dark secret. Perhaps it is simply the combination of all these things, plus its unmistakable cocoa aroma and sheer melt-in-the-mouth pleasure. Mmmmmmmm!

A little of what you crave for? But just because chocolate is so delightful, does not mean you should automatically feel guilty about having some. When you crave chocolate, or sugary, starchy, fatty or salty things, it is probably because your brain chemistry is missing something. The craving is a natural biological drive to restore the calmness and serenity that comes from a healthy balance of brain chemicals. In other words, your brain is trying to tell you that it wants a quick fix.

But a quick fix does not have to mean an overdose. Just a little of what you crave for can go a long way. One chocolate biscuit can do the trick. All it takes is a little chocolate, sugar, starch or fat to straighten out your turbulent brain.

So how can Lisa control her constant need for more chocolate? Can sheer will-power conquer it?

Sarah, aged 29, sees little hope of that:

The worst thing is being told to show some restraint and have some will power. It would be like saying to a heroin addict 'there's a cupboard full of heroin in the kitchen but you mustn't touch it'!

Rachel, aged 24, is pretty sceptical too:

Why stick at one bar, when you can have a dozen?

But you **can** resist the temptation to binge if you remember a few things:

- *one sweet or chocolate treat will trigger the feelgood chemicals just as quickly and powerfully as ten.*
- *quantity is not what you* really *want. You want the pleasure. You want it now. And you want it again. The more slowly you eat your treat, the more you can prolong the pleasure without feeling guilty, and the less likely you are to get the 'sugar dumps'.*
- *if you have something starchy beforehand, you'll find it much easier to resist the temptation to finish the packet.*

Stodge – craving-buster extraordinary
In exactly the same way that sugar cravings can be eased by a starchy meal or snack before the danger time, so too can chocolate cravings. Many dieters have discovered that a chunky sandwich, jacket potato or pasta midday meal can prevent the mid-afternoon cravings.

> **I find that simply by increasing the starches in my diet (pasta, rice, pulses, baked potatoes, baked beans, etc), I can greatly relieve my dreadful mood swings and chocolate cravings.**
>
> *Julie, aged 28*

This important serotonin-boosting, mood-lifting and craving-busting effect of starchy high-carbohydrate meals and snacks, especially in the premenstrual phase, is a key feature of the Body-clock Diet.

No forbidden foods

Strict taboo foods invite disaster because sooner or later you give in, hate yourself for being so pathetically weak-willed, throw away the diet plan, and gorge your way through the rest of the fridge.

Much better to have no forbidden foods – and allow yourself to have anything **in moderation**. If you weaken and eat one treat too many, do not tell yourself you have failed. Instead think of it as a little hiccup, a temporary setback, which you can soon recover from by being a little stronger next time – and keep persevering with the diet.

One of the great advantages of the Body-clock Diet is that it lets you indulge your food cravings – up to a point. In the premenstrual week you can have some chocolate treats when you want them – although not perhaps in the quantity you want them!

The Body-clock Diet responds to the rhythms of your mind and body, adapts to your changing moods, and helps you learn how to control your comfort food impulses.

But first, let us ask a few questions to find out just how rhythmic you really are – and when to harness the power of starchy food to keep your spirits up and your temptations down.

Chapter 5

Know Your Own Body-clock

Before you start the Body-clock Diet, you may find it helpful to know a little more about your own personal rhythms, so that you can choose the right alternatives that the diet has to offer at different times of the day, month and year.

Here is a simple biorhythm self-assessment quiz...

1. Do you have fairly regular periods?

YES – (score 3)
NO – (score 1)

If NO, please go to Question 3

2. If YES, how many days is the usual length of your complete cycle (from the first day of one period to the first day of the next)?

21 days or more – (score 3)
20 days or less – (score 1)

Please go to Question 4

3. If NO, how do they vary?

Usually 25 days or more – (score 3)
Usually 24 days or less – (score 1)
No clear pattern – (score 0)

4. Do you usually experience a mood change at a particular time of your cycle?

YES – (score 3)
NO – (score 0)

If NO, please go to question 7

5. If YES, when do you feel at your lowest or most irritable? (tick one only)

Just after your period? – (score 0)
Around mid-cycle? – (score 1)
From around mid-cycle until your period? – (score 3)
In the few days leading up to your period? – (score 3)
During your period? – (score 1)
Some other time? – (score 0)

6 Have you tried any of the following self-help treatments?

Evening Primrose Oil?:

YES and it helped a lot – (score 3)
YES and it helped a little – (score 1)
YES and it made no difference – (score 0)
NO – (score 1)

Vitamin B6?:

YES and it helped a lot – (score 3)
YES and it helped a little – (score 1)
YES and it made no difference – (score 0)
NO – (score 1)

Magnesium?:

YES and it helped a lot– (score 3)
YES and it helped a little – (score 1)
YES and it made no difference – (score 0)
NO – (score 1)

Any other self-help treatment (such as multivitamins, other minerals, herbal teas, Chinese medicines, homeopathic treatment, etc)?:

YES and it helped a lot – (score 3)
YES and it helped a little – (score 1)
YES and it made no difference – (score 0)
NO – (score 1)

7. Do you usually experience food cravings at a particular time of your cycle?

YES – (score 3)
NO – (score 0)

If NO, please go to question 11

8. If YES, when do you feel the cravings mostly?
(tick one only)

Just after your period? – (score 0)
Around mid-cycle? – (score 1)
From around mid-cycle until your period? – (score 3)
In the few days leading up to your period? – (score 3)
During your period? – (score 1)
Some other time? – (score 0)

9. What time of day do you feel cravings mostly?
(tick no more than two)

Early morning? – (score 0)
Mid morning? – (score 1)
Late morning? – (score 3)
Midday? – (score 1)
Early afternoon? – (score 3)
Mid afternoon? – (score 3)
Late afternoon? – (score 1)
Early evening? – (score 1)
Mid evening? – (score 1)
Late evening? – (score 3)
During the night? – (score 0)

10. What do you usually crave most?
(tick one only)

Chocolatey things? – (score 3)
Sweet things? – (score 3)
Starchy things? – (score 3)
Salty things? – (score 1)
Fatty things? – (score 1)
Something else? – (score 0)

11. Which is your main meal usually?

Breakfast? – (score 0)
Lunch (midday)? – (score 1)
Evening? – (score 3)
Some other time? – (score 0)

12. Do you find dieting difficult at a particular time of your cycle?

YES – (score 3)
NO – (score 0)

If NO, please go to Question 14

13. If YES, when is dieting most difficult?
(tick one only)

Just after your period? – (score 0)
Around mid-cycle? – (score 1)
From around mid-cycle until your period? – (score 3)
In the few days leading up to your period? – (score 3)
During your period? – (score 1)
Some other time? – (score 0)

14. By how much does your weight usually fluctuate (yo-yo) during a typical full menstrual cycle?

By less than 1 kg (2lb)? – (score 0)
By more than 1-3 kg (2-7lb)? – (score 1)
By more than 3 kg (7 lb)? – (score 3)

15. *Would you describe yourself as a 'lark' (brighter in the mornings) or 'owl' (brighter in the evenings) or neither?*

Lark – (score 3)
Owl – (score 1)
Neither – (score 0)

16. *Do you suffer at all from 'winter blues' (depressed mood in winter months)?*

YES definitely – (score 3)
YES a little – (score 1)
NO – (score 0)

Right, that's it. End of quiz.
Your answers will be useful in two ways.

Later on, when you embark on one of the Body-clock Diet plans, you may find it very helpful to refer back to them to help you decide:

- *when to switch from one phase of the plan to the next*
- *when to eat a more carbohydrate-boosted meal to lift your mood*
- *when to time your snacks to prevent cravings.*

The other use of the quiz is to tot up your scores and find out how well-suited you are for the Body-clock Diet.

Needless to say, it is only a rough-and ready guide

If you scored under 10: Your rhythms have relatively little effect on your mood, appetite, body chemistry or weight. But you will still find the Body-clock Diet an effective, healthy and different way of losing weight.

If you scored 10-19: Your rhythms are quite influential and could be playing a significant part in your attempt to lose weight. You could well benefit from the special features of the Body-clock Diet.

If you scored 20-39: Your rhythms play an important part in your moods, eating and metabolism. You should respond very well to the Body-clock Diet.

If you scored 40 or more: You have rhythm in your very bones! I cannot imagine how you have survived so far without the Body-clock Diet!

chapter 6

The Body-clock Diet Basics

So much for the theory. Let us get down to the basics of the Body-clock Diet itself.

In essence, it is a reduced fat, high carbohydrate eating plan to help you lose weight sensibly and safely. But, unlike other diets, it also has the remarkable feature of being specially designed to fit in with your menstrual cycle.

The diet that changes as YOU change
The Body-clock Diet is divided into three separate phases – A, B and C – each with a different dietary balance and calorie content to match your changing body chemistry during a complete menstrual cycle. To refresh your memory about the phases of the cycle, flick back to the brief description on page 24.

The essence is that **you start the diet during your period**, and then follow each phase of the diet, one after the other, according to the phase of your cycle, until your next period when you repeat the sequence.

This is how the diet changes with each phase of your cycle:

Phase A ('All right but Austere')
For most women this phase takes up the first fourteen days or so of the cycle, starting on Day 1 of your period or as soon as you are in the right frame of mind.

It is the most calorie-reduced phase – low in fatty and sugary things, but with plenty of fibre-rich starchy foods, vegetables and fruit. The low calorie content ensures that you lose weight well.

If you are on the Body-clock Exercise Programme you are allowed extra calories to help you through this phase.

Phase B ('Betwixt and Between')

This phase starts when your mood begins to change – for most women about ten to fourteen days before the period is due. It remains low fat but allows some sweet or starchy treats. The calorie content is increased a little ('B' is also for 'Better'!).

It may be a time of mood swings, but most women feel a more distinct change of mood a few days before their period, becoming a little more tense or even tearful, and perhaps getting cravings for chocolate, sweet things, salty or fatty things. This is the time to switch to Phase C of the plan.

Phase C ('Craving for Comfort')

This is usually confined to the last week of your cycle – often just the few days before the period when your mood is lowest and cravings worst.

In this phase the diet allows three starchy or sugary snacks or treats, including chocolate – so the calorie allowance is relatively generous. For this reason the length of this phase should be kept to a minimum.

Even so, you will still be losing body fat although you may gain a little weight because of fluid retention. In our two-cycle trial, there was a net loss of weight each month, averaging 4.4 kg (9.8 lb) (including 'phantom fat').

Switching phases

You can either switch from one phase to the next according to your mood or feelings, or, if you have a more-or-less regular 28-day virtually trouble-free cycle with just a few premenstrual days, you can arrange the diet on a simple week-by-week rota, starting with the first day of your period, like this:

Week 1: Start Phase A
Week 2: Continue Phase A
Week 3: Switch to Phase B
Week 4: Switch to Phase C

Dietary Phases of a Typical Cycle

Needless to say, the longer you can keep to the more calorie-reduced phases, A and B, the more quickly you will lose weight.

If your cycle is not exactly twenty-eight days, you can easily adjust the diet (see page 62 for details). For instance, if your cycle is nearer five weeks long you would usually have a longer Phase A – perhaps lasting up to about twenty-one days. And if your cycle is only three weeks long, you may spend little over a week in Phase A.

Three plans in one

To ensure that, as well as matching your cycle, it also matches your weight loss requirements, the Body-clock Diet has been formulated as three different eating plans according to the daily calorie intake best suited to you, averaged over the whole cycle:

- *a 1000 calorie a day plan (Plan 1000)*
- *a 1250 calorie a day plan (Plan 1250)*
- *a 1500 calorie a day plan (Plan 1500)*

Plan 1000 is intended for women with least weight to lose. Plan 1500 for those with most to lose. This may sound the wrong way round to you but it actually makes good sense, and conforms with the latest expert recommendations. It has nothing to do with how quickly you want to lose weight – this should be at about the same rate for all three plans if selected correctly. Instead it's based on your metabolic rate and is calculated to avoid triggering the 'famine response' and causing a plateau.

It's a surprising fact that the more overweight you are, the **higher** your metabolic rate (energy 'tickover' speed) – heavier people burn up calories faster. This means that, to lose weight satisfactorily, you **do not** need to restrict your calorie intake quite as much as someone who is less overweight than you.

A little further on, I shall describe how to select the right plan for yourself based on your starting weight. But remember that, as you succeed in losing weight, you may find yourself progressing from one plan to another – for example, from Plan 1250 to Plan 1000. Simply join the new plan at the next Phase A.

An easy diet to follow
The value of the Body-clock Diet, is that it is very simple and straightforward, as you will discover when you look through this book and get to know it a little better.

...and it's ultra-healthy too!
The overall nutritional balance of the Body-clock Diet is in line with the World Health Organization's most recent recommendations, and follows the same principles as the much-praised and much-relished Mediterranean way of eating – healthy and delicious.

More than half the calories in the Body-clock Diet come from satisfying starchy foods like potatoes, bread, rice and pasta, and each day includes at least five portions of fruit and vegetables, packed with health-giving antioxidant A,C, and E vitamins and important minerals. Only about 25-30 per cent of the calories in the Body-clock Diet come from fat.

Share it with the family
You will find the menus and recipes too enticing to keep to yourself – so why not share them with the family? They can always have larger portions and more extras if they want. Most of the recipes in Chapter 10

are calculated to serve four slimmers equally – but the three other slimmers' portions can easily be adjusted to feed one non-slimming husband and two starving children!

More than just a diet

The Body-clock Diet is not just a slimming diet. It also comes with two additional elements which experience has shown are crucial for successful and lasting weight loss:

- *The Body-clock Exercise Programme: graded exercises and activities which you can adapt to your needs throughout the month.*
- *The Body-clock StaySlim Plan: a scientifically-based plan that helps you to keep your new slimmer figure.*

The Body-clock Diet Basic Steps

The theory behind the Body-clock Diet may sound rather complicated – but the steps are very simple:

STEP 1 Decide how much to lose
     (using the chart below)
STEP 2 Select the right plan
     (and exercise programme)
STEP 3 Time it right
STEP 4 Suit yourself
STEP 5 Measure your progress

Let's take those steps one by one....

Step 1: Decide how much to lose

You may already have a very clear idea of this. You may, for instance, have decided that you want to lose a stone or three stone or whatever you feel is necessary. You may want to get back to what you used to weigh last summer, or the summer before that, or perhaps the sylph-like creature you were before you started your family.

That's fine, as long as you're being realistic and not setting yourself an impossible goal. If you have any doubts about this, check yourself using the chart on the next page.

Down to target...

If you don't yet know your target weight, or how much you should try to lose, then the chart will show you what weight is regarded as 'desirable' for your height. In fact, what the chart provides is a target weight range for each height (shown by the band labelled 'Target'), and you can choose from within that range.

Usually, if you're relatively 'large-framed' (wide-hipped or 'big-boned') it's best to choose a target at the heavier end of the range. If you're 'small-framed' (narrow-hipped), try for the lighter end of the target range.

But bear in mind that these are average figures – they may not necessarily be right for you. You may have inherited a body type that makes the 'normal' range just too unrealistic (see page 13) – and trying to reach it may cause a lot of unnecessary heartache.

...or in easy stages

But if you have a lot to lose, and you feel that reaching the normal 'Target' band all in one go is a bit too much to ask for, then set yourself a less demanding part-way target, and do your slimming in easy stages – slim, hold steady, slim, hold steady, slim, hold steady, and so on.

Step 2: Select the right plan

Check your present weight on the chart overleaf using the instructions on page 57 to find out the most suitable plan for you – Plan 1000, Plan 1250 or Plan 1500.

What's Your Plan?

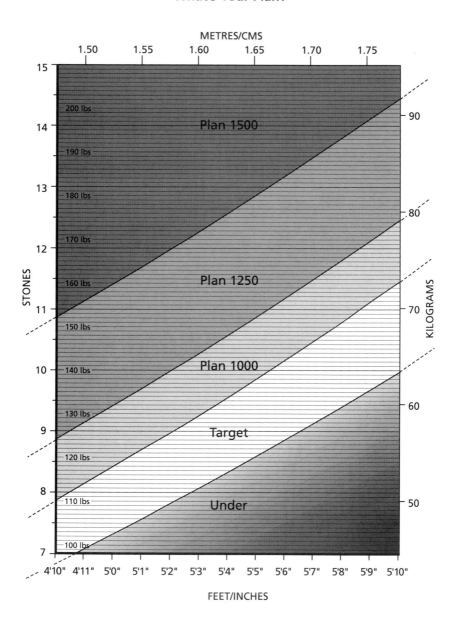

What's Your Plan?

To find your target weight...
1. First locate your height (without shoes) on either of the horizontal scales
   – metric or imperial, whichever's easier for you.
2. Now, using a ruler, or your finger as a guide, cast your eye vertically up the
   chart until it reaches the zone marked target. By looking horizontally
   across the chart you can read the weight that corresponds to the upper
   (and lower) limit of the target zone for your height. For example, if your
   height is 5'4", the upper limit of your target weight range is 9 st 8 1lb

To find the Body-clock Plan most suitable for you...
1. First locate your present weight on either of the vertical scales – metric
   or stones/pounds, whichever's easier for you.
2. Now run your finger horizontally across the chart until you meet the
   vertical line for your height. The zone in which these lines cross each
   other tells you which plan to follow. For example, if you're 5'4" and
   you currently weigh 11st 7lb, the two lines cross each other in the plan
   1250 zone.
3. Needless to say, as your weight comes down, the crossover point will
   move from one zone to another. For example, if you're 5'4" and you've
   been following Plan 1250, when you get down to 10 st 8 lb you should
   switch to Plan 1000. Similarly, when you get down to 8 st 9 lb you
   have reached the middle of your target zone and you could switch to
   the StaySlim plan.

The Three Plans
*Plan 1000 is best if you are less than 6.5 kg (1 stone) above
   target. It averages 1000 calories a day over the whole cycle
   and is quite a strict slimming diet.*
*Plan 1250 is best if you are anything from 6.5 to 20 kg
   (1 to 3 stones) above target. It averages 1250 calories a day –
   typical for a moderate slimming diet.*
*Plan 1500 is best if you need to lose over 20 kg (3 stones). It
   gives you a much gentler 1500 calories a day on average.*

Step 3: Time it right

It is important to start Phase A of the plan either on Day 1 of your cycle (first day of your period) or a day or two after – as soon as you feel in the right frame of mind for it.

Weigh yourself at this time and record the weight on your Weight-loss Progress Chart (see opposite).

Switch from one phase to the next according to the guidelines on pages 50-52. With a typical 28-day cycle, Phase A should last for about two weeks, the Phase B about one week and Phase C about one week. With Plan 1000, you should always switch from Phase A to Phase B after two weeks, whatever your mood.

Step 4: Suit yourself

Each day you will be offered choices of breakfasts, light meals and main meals from the menu lists. You should select one of each, although what time of day you eat these is up to you. You will also be offered Allowances, Ad Libs, Healthy Xtras, and Wicked Treats according to the Diet Rules on page 63.

Menu options

For the main meals, each phase of the plan offers not only a choice of different set menus and recipes – *Cook's Choice* – but also, in case you are too short of time or don't want to fiddle about too much, suggestions for something easier and simpler – *No-Fuss*.

As well as this choice, each phase of the plan also indicates the *vegetarian* menu options.

But remember, it's most important that you only select menu options from whichever phase of the plan you are currently going through. Never 'mix' phases.

Extras for exercise

If you're following the Body-clock Exercise Programme (see Chapter 11) you can add a 250-calorie extra for every 30 minutes of moderately vigorous activity – such as aerobics, skipping, running or swimming lengths. For example, the High Intensity programme allows you an extra 250 calories-worth a day. Select any item from the Healthy Xtras 250 list on page 67.

Weight-loss Progress Chart

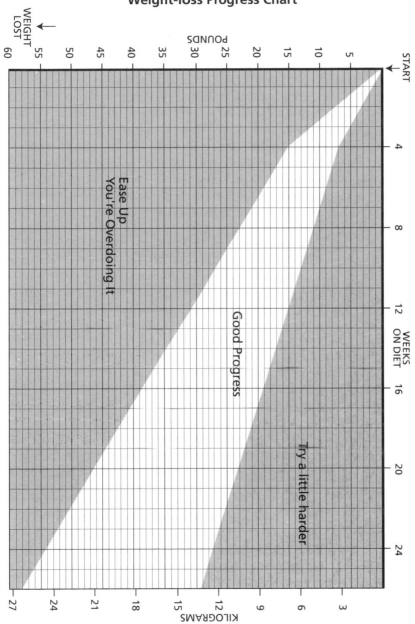

START

WEIGHT LOST

POUNDS

60 55 50 45 40 35 30 25 20 15 10 5

WEEKS ON DIET

4   8   12   16   20   24

KILOGRAMS

27 24 21 18 15 12 9 6 3

Ease Up
You're Overdoing It

Good Progress

Try a little harder

Step 5: Measure your progress

Do not weigh yourself more than once a week, however tempted you are to do so. Remember, your weight is meant to fluctuate throughout the month so only compare it with what it was **at the same time of your previous cycle.** The most important weighing is the first one after your period (on Day 1 or 2 of Phase A). A 'month-by-month' (cycle-by-cycle) graph of these weighings will show you your true weight-loss progress.

Do'nt be fooled by 'phantom fat'

Remember that your first weight loss is water, and that you will put the weight straight back on again when you stop dieting (see page 12). Make allowances for this in deciding whether or not you've reached your target.

No speeding

Don't try to lose too much, too quickly. Remember what we said about why so many other diets fail. If your calorie intake is less than the average recommended for your present weight band, then you are very likely to trigger the dreaded 'famine response' and hit a demoralizing plateau. Before you know what has happened, you'll break the diet and your weight will zoom skywards again.

This is why slimming experts recommend that you aim to lose about 450 to 900g (1-2 lb) a week (after the first week or two's 'phantom fat' loss). Yes it's slow – but it's steady.

Keeping motivated

It is no good dieting half-heartedly. Sticking to the rules, guidelines or recipes requires will-power. You must really want to succeed, and you must make yourself make the effort. There are no magic diets that can do this for you.

Of course, some diets can help you more than others – and the Body-clock Diet is certainly one of these, particularly at those times when your will-power is most likely to flag. But the big success-factor is you. You, and only you, can make the real difference between a diet that works for you and a diet that doesn't.

So, do whatever you can to convince yourself that when you say you want to lose weight, you really mean it. Here are a few suggestions that have worked wonders for other slimmers:

- *Remind yourself of your main reasons for losing weight – for example: to get in shape for the beach or some special occasion; to look good in smart clothes; to be fitter and healthier.*
- *Find a photo of yourself in your overweight state, and pin it up near your bathroom mirror or the fridge as a reminder of what you are trying to escape from.*
- *Write a brief contract note with a trusted friend or loved one, promising to continue with the diet for 'x' weeks, or to lose at least 'y' in weight.*
- *Offer yourself a big reward for success: that longed-for holiday; an outing to your favourite show; the item of furniture you've always wanted; a complete make-over or new outfit.*
- *Take each day, each meal, one at a time. Do not look ahead to weeks, months or years of dieting.*
- *Think of your diet as sensible eating principles that you have chosen to follow, rather than a strict diet that you have saddled yourself with.*
- *Do not give up just because you have 'broken' your diet and pigged out on something 'wicked'. Put it down to a temporary setback, and carry on as before.*
- *Be positive. Tell yourself you CAN succeed, and you WILL succeed.*

Some questions answered
Here are some of the questions you may wish to ask about the Body-clock Diet.

What if my cycle is not exactly 28 days?
No problem. The Body-clock Diet can usually be quite easily adjusted to fit your own cycle. You can even use it if your periods are quite irregular.

The simplest way to do this is to let your mind and body be your guide. As soon as you feel yourself changing in the second half of your cycle – perhaps becoming a bit moody or having more of an appetite – switch first to Phase B of the plan. And then, if you begin to feel clearly premenstrual – for example, edgy, bloated or tearful – switch into Phase C. Only when you have started your period and you are your normal self again should you return to Phase A.

For instance, if your cycle is nearer five weeks long you would usually have a longer Phase A – perhaps lasting up to about twenty-one days. And if your cycle is only three weeks long, you may spend little over a week in Phase A.

If you usually go straight from feeling perfectly okay to feeling thoroughly premenstrual, then switch your diet directly from Phase A to Phase C. But remember, the fewer 'C' days you have, the more quickly you will lose weight.

There may be some months when you don't notice any change from one period to the next – in which case you can simply carry on with Phase A or B all the way through.

What if I don't feel like starting on Day 1 of my period?
No problem. You don't have to start then. The best time to start is as soon as your premenstrual (or menstrual) symptoms have faded enough for you to feel reasonably positive about yourself again, which may not be until two or three days into your period, perhaps longer.

But it's important not to leave the start much later than that because you want to try to have as many 'A' days as possible.

What if I'm on the Pill?
You should find the diet even easier to follow because the Pill helps to keep your cycle regular.

What if I get pregnant?
Stop dieting straight away. Instead, eat a satisfying and healthy variety of foods, providing an abundance of major nutrients, including protein, vitamins and minerals. Stop smoking, cut right down on alcohol, and book yourself in for antenatal care.

But keep up with your exercises or other physical activity – you will soon need as much stamina, strength, suppleness and sparkle as you can muster!

And if I'm on HRT?

The Body-clock Diet is not really suitable for women who are going through the menopause. This is because your periods usually become so irregular or infrequent that the phases of the diet may be too difficult to follow. Needless to say, once your periods stop altogether, the rhythmic aspect of the diet ceases to apply. However, you can still derive the benefit of a low fat, healthy balanced slimming diet simply by sticking to Phase B continuously.

Some women in their forties may be prescribed HRT even though they are still having fairly regular periods and their menopause has not yet begun, in which case there is no reason why they should not follow the Body-clock Diet.

Is there anyone else the Body-clock Diet is NOT suitable for?

You should not go on **any** slimming diet if:
- *you're trying to conceive, or you're breastfeeding*
- *you're susceptible to an eating disorder such as bulimia or anorexia*
- *you're under 18*

And it's best to ask your doctor first if:
- *you have, or have ever had, a serious medical problem*
- *you're worried about any other aspect of your health.*

The Body-clock Diet rules

The following basic rules apply whichever plan you're on. If a plan differs in any respect, details are given in the introductory remarks to that plan.

- *Each day choose one 'breakfast', one 'light meal' and one 'main meal'. It's up to you precisely what time of day you eat each meal – for instance, you may want 'breakfast' mid-morning or the 'main meal' in the middle of the day or in the evening. But space them well apart.*

- *In Phase C of the plan you're encouraged to have three snacks/treats a day in addition to your set meals. Again it's up to you when you take these. Most women choose a mid-morning 'coffee-time' snack, a mid-afternoon 'tea-time' snack, and a late-night 'bed-time' snack.*

- *Your Phase C snacks/treats should preferably be starchy carbohydrate foods to help prevent cravings, but it's up to you. Choose the items you want from the Healthy Xtras or Wicked Treats lists up to, but no more than, the specified amounts. Also, remember that, as far as alcohol is concerned, the current medical advice for women is to refrain from drinking more than fourteen 'units' a week. A unit is one glass of wine, 300 ml (½ pint) of ordinary strength beer, lager or cider, one pub measure of sherry, vermouth or liqueur, or one single shot of gin, vodka, whisky, brandy or rum.*

- *It's important to vary your choices from day to day to get a wide variety of nutrients.*

- *Always keep to choices selected from the range offered for whichever phase you happen to be in. Do not 'mix' phases.*

- *Keep to the weights and measurements shown. This is especially important with anything oily or fatty. An extra teaspoon of these can really push up the calories so don't guess. It's not so crucial with high-fibre starchy staples, and even less so with vegetables or fruit.*

- *For vegetables, weights given are uncooked. Steaming or boiling does not appreciably alter calorie value.*

- *With meat, remove all visible fat before cooking. Grill rather than fry. With casseroles, gravies and sauces, pour off any surplus fat first.*

- *If you do fry anything, use sunflower oil, olive oil, corn oil, or safflower oil which are high in polyunsaturates and healthier for the heart. Avoid 'blended vegetable oil' or lard.*

Allowances

- *Milk: in addition to the milk, yoghurt or fromage frais in the meals, you're allowed an extra 300 ml (½ pint) skimmed OR 200 ml (7 fl oz) semi-skimmed milk a day. Alternatively (instead of milk), 2 x 125 g (5 oz) cartons of diet yoghurt or 2 x 100 g (4 oz) pots of low-fat fromage frais. This 'milk' allowance (about 100 calories) ensures you get enough calcium.*
- *Salad: In addition to the choices, eat a generous 'free' mixed vegetable salad each day (from the Ad Lib list below), with oil-free dressing, either with a meal or as a snack.*
- *Fruit: In addition to the choices, eat 100 calories-worth of fruit a day, selected from the Healthy Xtras 100 list below.*

Ad libs

Have as much as you like of the following:

- *Unlimited amounts of water, diet soft drinks, unsugared coffee or tea (using milk from your allowance), herbal tea, beef tea, yeast extract or other clear savoury drink. However, remember that beef tea, yeast extract and many other savoury drinks have a high salt content.*
- *Virtually unlimited quantities of: lettuce, tomato, cucumber, celery, cress, radish, beansprouts, onion (including pickled), garlic, chicory, cauliflower, courgettes, peppers, mushrooms, cabbage, carrot, spring greens and spinach. All either raw (with oil-free dressing if in a salad) or steamed and served hot.*
- *Unlimited amounts of herbs and spices.*
- *Artificial sweeteners.*

Healthy Xtras 100

Each item (•) below amounts to about 100 calories (for example, you can have five satsumas for 100 calories):

Fruit:
- *1 medium banana.*
- *2 x ½ an average-sized grapefruit.*
- *2 slices honeydew melon.*
- *2 rings fresh or canned (in juice) pineapple.*

- *2 medium apples, pears, oranges or peaches.*
- *5 satsumas.*
- *100 g (4 oz) semi-dried apricots.*
- *1 x 250 ml (8 fl oz) carton of long-life fruit juice.*

Starchy things:
- *1 wholewheat bisk OR 1 standard shredded wheat, plus 100 ml (3½ fl oz) skimmed milk.*
- *1 medium slice wholemeal bread, plus ⅓ of a small banana mashed as a spread.*
- *2 x rye crispbreads spread with 1 tbsp diet coleslaw.*
- *1 medium slice wholemeal bread, toasted; smear of low-fat spread; smear of yeast extract.*
- *1 medium slice wholemeal bread, toasted, covered with 2 tablespoons baked beans.*
- *1 mini-pitta bread smeared with 15 g (½ oz) houmous.*

Other:
- *150 g (5½ oz) natural low-fat yoghurt plus 1 teaspoon honey.*
- *2 x 100 g (4 oz) low fat fromage frais fruit flavours.*
- *125 g (5 oz) low fat fruit yoghurt plus a rich tea biscuit.*

Wicked treats 100
Each item (•) amounts to about 100 calories (for example, one 25 g (1 oz) bag of peanuts):

Tea-time things:
- *2 x shortbread, ginger nut, rich tea or butter crunch biscuits.*
- *1½ bourbons, chocolate chip cookies or custard creams.*
- *1 x 25 g (1 oz) bag peanuts.*
- *1 medium slice wholemeal bread, low-fat spread, smear of honey or jam.*

Chocolatey things:
- *two-fifths of a 50 g (2 oz) bar of plain, milk or white chocolate*
- *1 chocolate digestive biscuit.*
- *2 chocolate-topped orange cake-biscuits.*

Alcohol:
- *1 x 150 ml (5 fl oz) glass dry or medium white, red or rosé wine.*
- *1 x 300 ml (½ pint) ordinary strength lager, beer or cider.*
- *2 x 300 ml (½ pint) low-alcohol lager, beer or cider.*
- *1 medium-sized schooner sherry, port or madeira.*
- *1 pub measure sweet vermouth.*
- *2 x pub measures dry vermouth.*
- *2 x singles (or 1 double) gin, whisky, brandy, vodka, rum or tequila (with calorie-free mixer optional).*
- *1 pub measure liqueur or speciality drink.*

Healthy Xtras 250

Each item (•) below amounts to about 250 calories (for example, you can have twelve satsumas for 250 calories):

Fruit:
- *2 x large bananas.*
- *3 x small bananas.*
- *5 x medium apples, pears, oranges, or peaches.*
- *12 x satsumas.*
- *250 g (10 oz) semi-dried apricots.*
- *3 x 200 ml (7 fl oz) cartons long-life fruit juice.*

Starchy things:
- *50 g (2 oz) most breakfast cereals plus 150 ml (¼ pint) skimmed milk.*
- *1 wholemeal pitta bread, warmed, with 50 g (2 oz) houmous and 6 stoned black olives (in brine).*
- *2 medium slices of wholemeal bread, toasted, plus 150 g (5½ oz) baked beans.*
- *2 medium slices wholemeal bread, low-fat spread, and 1 small banana, sliced or mashed.*
- *40 g (1½ oz) bran flakes, 150 ml (¼ pint) skimmed milk, 1 small banana, chopped.*
- *1 x 65 g (2½ oz) wholemeal bap or muffin, toasted and covered with 50 g (2 oz) low-fat soft cheese; cucumber slices ad lib.*

Wicked treats 250

Each item (•) amounts to about 250 calories (for example, 3 x 25 g (1 oz) bags of peanuts). Mix and match as you wish.

Tea-time things:
- *5 x shortbread, gingernut, rich tea, or butter crunch biscuits.*
- *4 x bourbon, chocolate chip cookie, or custard cream biscuits.*
- *3 x 25 g (1 oz) bag peanuts.*
- *2 medium slices wholemeal toast, low-fat spread, and honey or jam (1 level tablespoon).*
- *1 x 75 g (3 oz) jam doughnut.*
- *75 g (3 oz) slice of cake (e.g. lemon or chocolate sponge, battenberg, swiss roll, rich fruit).*

Chocolatey things:
- *1 only of any 50 g (2 oz) plain, milk or white chocolate bar or packet, including chocolate caramel/toffee bars.*
- *1½ flaky chocolate bars.*
- *2 milky-filled chocolate bars.*
- *2 large chocolate waferbiscuits.*
- *2 chocolate orange 'club' biscuits.*
- *3 chocolate digestive biscuits.*
- *5 chocolate-topped orange cake-biscuits.*

Alcohol:
Note: Remember the medical advice is to refrain from drinking more than fourteen 'units' of alcohol per week. See page 64 at the mfor details.
- *2 x 150 ml (5 fl oz) glasses dry or medium white, red or rosé wine.*
- *2 x 300 ml (½ pint) ordinary strength beer or cider.*
- *5 x 300 ml (½ pint) low-alcohol lager or beer.*
- *4 x small glasses sherry, port or madeira.*
- *2 x pub measures sweet vermouth.*
- *4 x pub measures dry vermouth.*
- *4 x singles gin, whisky, vodka, rum, tequila (with calorie-free mixer optional).*
- *2 x pub measures liqueurs speciality drinks.*

Body-clock Plan 1000

About this plan

This Body-clock Diet plan provides about 1000 calories a day, averaged over a typical menstrual cycle. This is the plan to follow if you have less than one stone to lose in order to reach your target weight. The reason why slimmers with more to lose are allowed more calories is explained on page 53.

Plan 1000 is designed to be a short, sharp diet – but you will still find it surprisingly satisfying, with plenty of variety and delicious recipes. Most women who start their slimming with this plan can expect to lose up to 5lb in the first week, slightly less in the second week, and 1-2lb a week after that. So, hopefully, you should reach your target within one or two cycles, depending on exactly how much you want to lose. But remember, a few of those lost pounds will be 'phantom' ones – in other words, water (see page 12).

Menu options

For the main meals, each phase of the plan offers not only a choice of different set menus and recipes – '**Cook's Choice**' – but also, in case you're too short of time or don't want to fiddle about too much, suggestions for something easier and simpler – '**No-Fuss**'.

As well as this choice, each phase of the plan also indicates the vegetarian menu options (marked Ⓥ).

But remember, it's most important that you select only menu options from whichever phase of the plan you're currently going through. Never 'mix' phases.

Here we go...

Plan 1000 – Step by step

1 Before you start, make sure you're familiar with the BASIC STEPS outlined on pages 54-61 and the DIET RULES on pages 63-65.

2 Start the plan at the beginning of your Phase A. Remember that this is the most slimming phase – only 900 calories a day – so don't delay starting for too long otherwise you may not be able to cover your full fourteen days before you need to switch to the more calorific Phase B.

3 Don't forget that, if you're following the Body-clock Exercise Programme (see Chapter 11), you can add a 250 calorie extra for every 30 minutes of moderately vigorous activity – such as aerobics, skipping, running or swimming lengths. For example, the High Intensity programme allows you an extra 250 calories-worth a day. Select any item from the Healthy Xtras 250 list on page 67.

4 Unlike the other two Body-clock plans, which leave it to you to decide when to switch to Phase B, with Plan 1000 you are recommended not to stay in Phase A for more than 14 days. This is because the low calorie allowance of Phase A is likely to trigger the 'famine response' if continued any longer (see page 13).

5 Phase B gives you 1000 calories a day and the longer you can stay in it the better. You are allowed 100 calories-worth of extras, preferably from the Healthy Xtras 100 list. Phase B may last right up to your next period. But if you get severe cravings, you may have to switch to the Phase C.

6 Phase C, usually the last few days of your cycle, is different in several ways. It gives you:
   • more food (increased to about 1300 calories a day)
   • more often (six meals/snacks a day)
   • more carbohydrate to beat the cravings
   Because of the more generous calorie allowance during this phase, you should only switch to it if you feel the need – otherwise you will slow down your weight loss unnecessarily.

7 Once you have reached your target, the guidelines in Chapter 12 will help you adjust your calorie intakes to maintain your new slim weight.

Plan 1000 Menus

Make sure you select only from the choices specified in each phase of the plan.

Plan 1000 – PHASE A *(averaging about 900 cals/day)*

1000
A

Each day:
- select one breakfast, one light meal and one main meal;
- plus 'milk' from allowance (see page 65);
- plus 100 calories-worth of 'fruit' from Healthy Xtras 100 list (see page 65);
- plus Ad Lib salad, etc. *(see page 65).*

Phase A Breakfasts *(about 100 calories)*
Make sure you don't skip breakfast – it's not much but it helps you through the morning. Each day, pick any ONE of the following. Vary your choice from day to day:
- 25 g (1 oz) branflakes or standard shredded wheat; milk from allowance; fruit from allowance.
- 1 medium slice wholemeal bread, toasted; smear of low-fat spread; smear of yeast extract. Fruit from allowance.
- Fruit salad in 150 ml (¼ pint) apple juice; pick any two of:1 medium apple, 1 medium pear, 1 medium orange, 1 medium peach.
- 125 g (5 oz) low-fat fruit yoghurt (any flavour) plus 1 rye crispbread and a smear of low-fat spread.
- 1 small banana mashed in 2 tablespoons of half cream.
- ½ medium grapefruit; plus 1 rye crispbread and a smear of low-fat spread.
- 1 thin slice wholemeal bread with 1 teaspoon low-fat spread and 1 teaspoon reduced-sugar marmalade or jam. Fruit from allowance.
- 100 g (4 oz) low-fat fromage frais plus 1 medium apple, pear, peach or orange chopped in.

- 1 wholewheat bisk with 100 ml (3½ fl oz) skimmed milk. Fruit from allowance.
- 5 medium mushrooms, sliced and lightly fried in 7.5 g (¼ oz) sunflower margarine in a non-stick pan; served on 1 thin slice of wholemeal toast.
- 100 g (4 oz) melon plus ½ muffin smeared with 1 teaspoon low-fat spread.
- 1 medium apple, cored and baked with a filling of 20 g (¾ oz) raisins, plus low-fat natural yoghurt from milk allowance.
- ½ medium grapefruit; plus 1 thin slice wholemeal toast smeared with 1 teaspoon low-fat spread and a streak of yeast extract.
- I boiled egg (size 3) with 1 rye crispbread smeared with low-fat spread.

1000
A

Phase A Light Meals *(about 250 calories)*
Each day, pick any ONE of the following. Vary your choice from day to day:

- 200 g (7 oz) jacket-baked potato, filled with 150 g (5½ oz) baked beans. Salad or fruit from allowance.
- 2 x medium slices wholemeal bread smeared with low-fat spread; 65 g (2½ oz) lean ham; thin smear mustard. Salad or fruit from allowance.
- 2 x reduced-fat chipolata sausages, grilled; plus 1 x 150 g (5½ oz) baked beans. Salad or fruit from allowance.
- 65 g (2½ oz) wholemeal bap or muffin, toasted and covered with 50 g (2 oz) low-fat soft cheese; unlimited cucumber slices. Salad or fruit from allowance.
- 200 g (7 oz) jacket-baked potato, filled with 100 g (4 oz) cottage cheese with or without fresh chives chopped on. Salad or fruit from allowance.
- 100 g (4 oz) cooked weight cold pasta shells mixed with 1 medium apple, chopped, and 50 g (2 oz) tuna (in brine, drained) and ½ medium red pepper, chopped small, all tossed in 1 tablespoon fat-free French dressing.
- 1 medium slice of wholemeal bread, toasted, plus 150 g (5½ oz) baked beans, topped with 1 medium (size 3) poached egg. Salad or fruit from allowance.

- 200 g (7 oz) jacket-baked potato, filled with 50 g (2 oz) tuna (in brine, drained) mixed with 1 small onion or shallot, chopped. Salad or fruit from allowance.
- 1 hard-boiled egg (size 3) mashed with 1 teaspoon low-fat mayonnaise, served on 1 medium-sized wholemeal bap smeared with 2 teaspoons low-fat sunflower spread; garnished with unlimited cress. Salad or fruit from allowance.
- 2 medium slices wholemeal toast, spread with 25 g (1 oz) smoked mackerel pâté, garnished with crisp lettuce and cucumber slices. Fruit from allowance.
- 300 ml (½ pint) canned thick vegetable soup sprinkled with 1 tbsp grated Parmesan (or Cheddar); plus 1 crusty roll. Fruit from allowance.
- 200 g (7 oz) jacket-baked potato, filled with 100 g (4 oz) small seedless grapes and topped with 100 g (4 oz) low-fat natural fromage frais.
- 1 wholemeal pitta bread, warmed, with 50 g (2 oz) houmous and 6 stoned black olives (in brine); plus salad of choice from allowance.
- 150 g (5½ oz) button mushrooms simmered in 1 tablespoon dry white wine, plus 1 tablespoon tomato puree and 1 teaspoon wholegrain mustard, served on two halves of a wholemeal muffin, halved and toasted.

Phase A Main Meals *(about 350 calories)*
Each day, pick any ONE complete meal from either the 'Cook's Choice' or 'No Fuss' lists (preferably something quite different from your light meal). Vary your choice from day to day.

'Cook's Choice' Menus
- *Turkey Stir-Fry* (see page 112) 1 serving;
  1 piece of fruit from allowance.
- *Stuffed Peppers* (see page 101) Ⓥ 1 serving;
  50 g (2 oz) piece Edam, Gouda or low-fat soft cheese and a cracker or rye crispbread.
- *Vegetable Moussaka* (see page 102) Ⓥ 1 serving;
  1 piece of fruit from allowance.

**1000
A**

- *Cheese and Pineapple Pizza* (see page103) Ⓥ 1 serving;
  65 g (2½ oz) low-fat fruit fromage frais.
- *Fish with Peppers* (see page 122) 1 serving;
  2-3 small new potatoes boiled;
  piece of fruit from allowance.
- *Red Pepper Pasta* (see page103) Ⓥ 1 serving;
  125 g (5 oz) low-fat fruit yoghurt.
- *Tuna and Egg Salad* with roll (see page123) 1 serving;
  125 g (5 oz) low-fat fruit yoghurt.
- *Sausage Hotpot* (see page 116) 1 serving;
  1 piece of fruit from allowance.
- *Bacon and Cauliflower Cheese Bake* (see page 120) 1 serving;
  125 g (5 oz) low-fat fruit yoghurt.
- *French Chicken Casserole* (see page121) 1 serving;
  25 g (1 oz) low-fat soft cheese on a rye crispbread.
- *Baked Bean Gratin* (see page 104) Ⓥ 1 serving;
  1 apple, pear, orange, peach or kiwifruit.
- *Stir-fried Chicken and Mixed Vegetables* (see page121) 1 serving;
  65 g (2½ oz) frozen low-fat chocolate mousse.
- *Spiced Chick Peas* (see page 104) Ⓥ 1 serving;
  150 g (5½ oz) low-fat yoghurt, with fruit from allowance.
- *Worcester Salmon Bake* (see page124) 1 serving;
  salad and fruit from allowance.
- *Chilli con Carne* (see page 118) 1 serving, plus:
  Fruit from allowance.
- *Satay Salad* (see page 108) Ⓥ 1 serving, plus:
  Spicy Oranges (see page 130).
- *Lamb and Potato Fry* (see page 116) 1 serving;
  65 g (2½ oz) fromage frais, any flavour.

'No Fuss' Menus (350 calories)
NOTE: Each of the following serves ONE slimmer only. Multiply quantities by four to serve two young children and one non-slimming adult as well as yourself.
- 100 g (4 oz) gammon rasher, grilled; plus 200 g (7 oz) jacket-baked potato filled with 25 g (1 oz) cottage cheese; plus 25 g (1 oz) frozen peas, boiled. Fruit from allowance.

1000 A

- 1 thick slice wholemeal toast, smeared with low-fat spread, covered with 150 g (5½oz) baked beans, and topped with 1 poached egg (size 3).
  Fruit from allowance.
- 100 g (4 oz) well-trimmed chump lamb or pork chop, grilled; plus 100 g (4 oz) potato, boiled; plus 100 g (4 oz) frozen broccoli or other vegetable, steamed or boiled.
  Fruit from allowance.
- Tuna and egg salad made from 1 gem lettuce broken in a bowl; tossed with 100g (4 oz) tuna (in brine, drained); 200 g (7 oz) cooked new potatoes, sliced; tomato; spring onions; watercress; 1 hard-boiled egg (size 3), quartered; 3 black olives; 2 tablespoons reduced-fat French dressing.
  125 g (5 oz) low-fat fruit yoghurt.
- Mushroom omelette: a few mushrooms chopped and lightly fried in 1 teaspoon butter plus 1tablespoon corn oil, add 2 eggs (size 3) whisked with a little skimmed or semi-skimmed milk, seasoning and chopped chives (dried or fresh). Serve with salad with oil-free dressing.
  Fruit from allowance.
- Lamb kebab made with 4 x 2.5 cm (1 in) cubes lean lamb; 1 rasher back bacon, well-trimmed and sliced; 1 small onion, quartered; 1 tomato, quartered; green pepper, cut into squares; plus 1tablespoon barbecue sauce. Serve with 200 g (7 oz) boiled rice or potatoes.
  Salad and fruit from allowance.
- Pea soup: 100 g (4 oz) frozen peas, 50 g (2 oz) chopped onions and 100 g (4 oz) chopped potatoes lightly fried in a non-stick pan with a little oil; add 150 ml (¼ pint) vegetable stock, 150 ml (¼ pint) skimmed milk, and a little dried mint. Bring to the boil and simmer for 15 minutes. Serve with a roll or pitta bread.
  Fruit from allowance.
- Grilled white fish: medium portion of haddock, cod, or other white fish, grilled or poached, served with 100 g (4 oz) boiled peas, 200 g (7 oz) boiled new potatoes and 1 tablespoon tartare sauce.
  Fruit from allowance.

1000
A

- Chopped tomato pasta: 100 g (4 oz) pasta, boiled; plus a sauce made from 200 g (7 oz) canned chopped tomatoes (with herbs if preferred), cooked in a little oil with ½ teaspoon sugar and black pepper.
  Serve with a green salad from allowance.
  1 apple, orange, pear or peach.
- Chicken and vegetable stir-fry: 1 skinned medium chicken breast, sliced into small cubes, stir-fried with beansprouts, mushrooms, mangetout or runner beans, herbs and spices to taste. Serve with 200 g (7 oz) boiled rice.
  Fruit from allowance.
- Cauliflower cheese: 175 g (6 oz) cauliflower florets, boiled, covered with a cheese sauce made with 50 g (2 oz) reduced-fat Cheddar, 1 tbsp cornflour and 175 ml (6 fl oz) skimmed milk. Grill in an ovenproof dish until bubbling. Green salad from allowance.
  4 ready-to-eat dried apricots or 1 small apple.
- 200 g (7 oz) jacket-baked potato, filled with 150 g (5½ oz) baked beans. Salad from allowance.
  1 apple, pear, orange or peach.
- 100 g (4 oz) cooked weight cold pasta shells mixed with 1 medium apple, chopped, and 50 g (2 oz) tuna (in brine, drained) and ½ red pepper, chopped; all tossed in 1 tbsp reduced-fat French dressing.
  125 g (5 oz) low-fat fruit yoghurt.
- 300 ml (½ pint) canned thick vegetable soup sprinkled with 1 tablespoon grated Parmesan or Cheddar, plus 1 crusty roll.
  1 apple, pear, orange or peach.

Phase A Snacks/Treats
NONE – Sorry! – but don't forget your 100 calorie fruit allowance (pick from the Healthy Xtras 100 list on page 65) and free mixed salad from the Ad Lib list also on page 65.

Plan 1000 – PHASE B *(averaging about 1000 cals/day)*

After the austerity of Phase A, things ease up a little in this 'B' for 'Better' phase. You are allowed an extra 100 calories-worth of snacks or treats in addition to the meals, allowances and ad libs.

1000 B

Phase B Breakfasts *(about 100 calories)*
Choose from the Phase A selection beginning on page 71.

Phase B Light Meals *(about 250 calories)*
Choose from the Phase A selection beginning on page 72.

Phase B Main meals *(about 350 calories)*
Choose from the Phase A selection beginning on page 73.

Phase B Snacks/Treats *(about 100 calories)*
Preferably something fruity or starchy from the Healthy Xtras 100 list on page 65. But you can choose from the Wicked Treats 100 list if you wish.

- Mix and match as you like, but remember the sensible limit for alcohol (see page 64).
- These extras are in addition to your usual allowances and ad libs (see page 65).

1000
C

Plan 1000 – PHASE C *(averaging about 1300 cals/day)*

This is the 'C' for 'Craving' phase, and, as you can see, it allows 3 x 100 calorie snacks or treats of your choice each day in addition to the meals, allowances and ad libs. You can use these snacks to help you through the cravings by choosing starchy, sugary, or chocolatey things if you like – as long as you keep to the limit.
Remember that the fewer days you spend in this phase of the plan, the faster will be your weight loss.

Phase C Breakfasts *(about 100 calories)*
Choose from the Phase A selection beginning on page 71.

Phase C Light Meals *(about 250 calories)*
Choose from the Phase A selection beginning on page 72.

Phase C Main Meals *(about 350 calories)*
Choose from the Phase A selection beginning on page 73.

Phase C Snacks/Treats *(about 300 calories)*
Select three extra 100-calorie items from either the Healthy Xtras 100 list or the Wicked Treats 100 list.
- Preferably choose starchy things to help ease the cravings – but of course the choice is yours.
- Mix and match as you like – but keep to the limit for each item, and remember the sensible limits for alcohol (see page 64).
- Use your answers to Question 9 of the 'Know Your Own Body-clock' quiz on page 47 to help decide what time of day to have your starchy snacks.
- You may prefer to bolster your meals with extras or space your snacks evenly throughout the day so that you never have too long to wait.
- Remember, these extras are in addition to your usual allowances and ad libs (see page 65).

chapter 8

Body-clock Plan 1250

About this plan

This Body-clock Diet plan provides about 1250 calories a day, averaged over a typical menstrual cycle. This is the plan to follow if you have between 1-3 stone to lose in order to reach your target weight. The reason why slimmers who have more to lose are allowed more calories is explained on page 53.

Plan 1250 is designed to be a medium term diet – surprisingly satisfying, with plenty of variety and delicious recipes. Most women in the above category who start their slimming with this plan can expect to lose up to 5lb in the first week, slightly less in the second week, and 1-2lb a week after that. So, hopefully, you should reach your target within two to five cycles, depending on exactly how much you want to lose. But remember, a few of those lost pounds will be 'phantom' ones – in other words water (see page 12).

Menu options

For the main meals, each phase of the plan offers not only a choice of different set menus and recipes – '**Cook's Choice**' – but in case you are too short of time or don't want to fiddle about too much, suggestions for something easier and simpler – '**No-Fuss**'.

As well as this choice, each phase of the plan also indicates the vegetarian menu options (marked Ⓥ).

But remember, it's most important that you select only menu options from whichever phase of the plan you are currently going through. Never 'mix' phases.

Here we go...

Plan 1250 – Step by step

1 Before you start, make sure you're familiar with the BASIC STEPS outlined on pages 54-61 and the DIET RULES on pages 63-65.

2 Start the plan at the beginning of your Phase A. Remember that Phase A is the most slimming phase – only 1000 calories a day – so don't delay starting for too long otherwise you may not be able to cover your full fourteen days before you find you need to switch to the more calorific Phase B.

3 Don't forget that, if you're following the Body-clock Exercise Programme (see Chapter 11), you can add a 250 calorie extra for every 30 minutes of moderately vigorous activity – such as aerobics, skipping, running or swimming lengths. For example, the High Intensity programme allows you an extra 250 calories-worth a day. Select any item from the Healthy Xtras 250 list on page 67.

4 It's best to switch to Phase B after about fourteen days. Continuing Phase A much beyond that may trigger the 'famine response' (see page 13).

5 Phase B gives you 1250 calories a day and the longer you can stay in it before switching to Phase C the better. You're allowed a bigger breakfast, a bigger light meal, and 100 calories-worth of extras or treats, preferably from the Healthy Xtras 100 list. Phase B may last right up to your next period. But if you get severe cravings, you may have to switch to Phase C.

6 Phase C, usually the last few days of the cycle, is different in several ways. It gives you:

   • more food (increased to about 1750 calories a day)
   • more often (six meals/snacks a day)
   • more carbohydrate to beat the cravings

   Because of the more generous calorie allowance during this phase, you should only switch to it if you feel the need – otherwise you will slow down your weight loss unnecessarily.

7 Once you have reached your target, the guidelines in Chapter 12 will help you adjust your calorie intakes to maintain your new slim weight.

Plan 1250 Menus

Make sure you select only from the choices specified for each phase of the plan.

Plan 1250 – PHASE A *(averaging about 1000 cals/day)*

Each day:
- 🍎 select one breakfast, one light meal and one main meal;
- 🍎 plus 'milk' from allowance (see page 65);
- 🍎 plus 100 calories-worth of fruit from Healthy Xtras 100 list (see page 65).
- 🍎 plus Ad Lib salad (see page 65).

1250 A

Phase A Breakfasts *(about 100 calories)*

Make sure you don't skip breakfast – it's not much but it helps you through the morning. Each day, pick any ONE of the following. Vary your choice from day to day:

- 25 g (1 oz) branflakes or standard shredded wheat; milk from allowance; fruit from allowance.
- 1 medium slice wholemeal bread, toasted; smear of low-calorie spread; smear of yeast extract. Fruit from allowance.
- Fruit salad in 150 ml (¼ pint) apple juice; pick any two of: 1 medium apple, 1 medium pear, 1 medium orange, 1 medium peach.
- 125 g (5 oz) low-fat fruit yoghurt (any flavour) plus 1 rye crispbread and a smear of low-fat spread.
- 1 small banana mashed in 2 tablespoons half cream.
- ½ medium grapefruit; plus 1 rye crispbread and a smear of low-fat spread.
- 1 thin slice wholemeal bread with 1 teaspoon low-fat spread and 1 teaspoon reduced-sugar marmalade or jam. Fruit from allowance.
- 100 g (4 oz) low-fat fromage frais plus 1 medium apple, pear, peach or orange chopped in.

- 1 wholewheat bisk with 100 ml (3½ fl oz) skimmed milk. Fruit from allowance.
- 5 medium mushrooms, sliced and lightly fried gently in 7.5 g (¼ oz) sunflower margarine in a non-stick pan; served on 1 thin slice of wholemeal toast.
- 100 g (4 oz) melon plus ½ muffin smeared with 1 teaspoon low-fat spread.
- 1 medium apple, cored and baked with a filling of 20 g (¾ oz) raisins, plus low-fat natural yoghurt from milk allowance.
- ½ medium grapefruit; plus 1 thin slice wholemeal toast smeared with 1 teaspoon low-fat spread and a streak of yeast extract.
- 1 boiled egg (size 3) with 1 rye crispbread smeared with low-fat spread.

Phase A Light Meals *(about 250 calories)*
Each day, pick any ONE of the following. Vary your choice from day to day:

1250
A

- 200 g (7 oz) jacket-baked potato, filled with 150 g (5½ oz) baked beans. Salad or fruit from allowance.
- 2 medium slices wholemeal bread smeared with low-fat spread; 65 g (2½ oz) lean ham; thin smear mustard. Salad or fruit from allowance.
- 2 reduced-fat chipolata sausages, grilled; plus 150 g (5½ oz) baked beans. Salad or fruit from allowance.
- 65 g (2½ oz) wholemeal bap or muffin, toasted and covered with 50 g (2 oz) low-fat soft cheese; unlimited cucumber slices. Salad or fruit from allowance.
- 200 g (7 oz) jacket-baked potato, filled with 100 g (4 oz) cottage cheese with or without fresh chives chopped on. Salad or fruit from allowance.
- 100 g (4 oz) cooked weight cold pasta shells mixed with 1 medium apple, chopped, and 50 g (2 oz) tuna (in brine, drained) and ½ medium red pepper, chopped small, all tossed in 1 tablespoon fat-free French dressing.
- 1 medium slice of wholemeal bread, toasted, plus 150 g (5½ oz) baked beans, topped with 1 poached egg (size 3). Salad or fruit from allowance.

- 200 g (7 oz) jacket-baked potato, filled with 50 g (2 oz) tuna (in brine, drained) mixed with 1 small onion or shallot, chopped. Salad or fruit from allowance.
- 1 hard-boiled egg (size 3) mashed with 1 teaspoon low-fat mayonnaise, served on 1 medium-sized wholemeal bap smeared with 2 teaspoons low-fat sunflower spread; garnished with unlimited cress. Salad or fruit from allowance.
- 2 medium slices wholemeal toast, spread with 25 g (1 oz) smoked mackerel pâté, garnished with crisp lettuce and cucumber slices. Fruit from allowance.
- 300 ml (½ pint) canned thick vegetable soup sprinkled with 1 tbsp grated Parmesan or Cheddar; plus 1 crusty roll. Fruit from allowance.
- 200 g (7 oz) jacket-baked potato, filled with 100 g (4 oz) small seedless grapes and topped with 100 g (4 oz) low-fat natural fromage frais.
- 1 wholemeal pitta bread, warmed, with 50 g (2 oz) houmous and 6 stoned black olives (in brine); plus salad of choice from allowance.
- 150 g (5½oz) button mushrooms simmered in 1 tablespoon dry white wine, plus 1 tablespoon tomato purée and 1 teaspoon wholegrain mustard, served on a wholemeal muffin, halved and toasted.

1250 A

Phase A Main Meals *(about 450 calories)*
Each day, pick any ONE complete meal from either the 'Cook's Choice' or 'No Fuss' lists (preferably something quite different from your light meal). Vary your choice from day to day.

'Cook's Choice' Menus
- *Ham and Prawn Jambalaya* (see page 113) 1 serving; Fruit and/or low-fat yoghurt from allowances.
- *Bacon and Potato Bake* (see page 115) 1 serving; Green salad from ad libs plus: 62 g (2½oz) frozen fruit mousse.
- *Spaghetti Bolognese* (see page 117) 1 serving; Green salad from ad libs; Fresh fruit and/or low-fat yoghurt from allowances.
- *Apricot Lamb Pilaf* (see page 119) 1 serving; Low-fat yoghurt from allowance.

- *Pork and Prunes* (see page119) 1 serving;
  150g (5½oz) new potatoes, boiled or baked,
  Green salad from ad libs,
  Low fat yoghurt from allowance.
- *Prawn and Mushroom Risotto* (see page 123) 1 serving;
  Salad from ad libs plus:
  1 apple, pear, orange or peach.
- *Pasta Stroganoff* (see page 105) Ⓥ 1 serving;
  Salad from ad libs plus:
  Low-fat natural or fruit yoghurt.
- *Eggs Florentine* (see page107) Ⓥ 1 serving;
  75 g (3 oz) new potatoes, boiled or baked.
  Fresh fruit or low-fat yoghurt from allowance.
- *Vegetable Casserole with Dumplings* (see page 106) Ⓥ 1 serving;
  Spicy Oranges (see page 130).
- *Spicy Bean Hot Pot* (see page 107) Ⓥ 1 serving;
  Green salad from ad libs plus:
  1 apple, pear, orange, or peach.
- *Sausage and Corn Cheese Muffins* (see page 110) 1 serving;
  Green salad from ad libs,
  1 apple, pear, orange or peach.
- *Turkey Two-Pepper Salad* (see page111) 1 serving;
  Low-fat natural or fruit yoghurt from allowance.
- *French Onion Soup* (see page 109) 1 serving;
  Pears in Wine Sauce (see page 129).
- *Crab Noodle Stir-Fry* (see page125) 1 serving;
  62 g (2½oz) frozen fruit mousse.

'No Fuss' Menus *(about 450 calories)*
NOTE: Each of the following serves ONE slimmer only. Multiply quantities by 4 to serve two young children and one non-slimming adult as well as yourself.
- 100 g (4 oz) gammon rasher, grilled; plus 200 g (7 oz) jacket-baked potato filled with 25 g (1 oz) cottage cheese; plus 25 g (1 oz) frozen peas, boiled.
  25 g (1 oz) slice low-fat cheese on a cracker or crispbread.
  Fruit from allowance.

1250 A

- 1 thick, large, slice wholemeal toast, smeared with low-fat spread, covered with 150 g (5½ oz) baked beans, and topped with 2 low-fat chipolata sausages and 1 poached egg (size 3).
  Fruit from allowance.
- 100 g (4 oz) well-trimmed chump lamb or pork chop, grilled; plus 100 g (4 oz) potato, boiled; plus 100g (4oz) frozen broccoli or other vegetable, steamed or boiled.
  25 g (1 oz) slice of low-fat cheese on a cracker or crispbread.
  Fruit from allowance.
- Tuna and egg salad made from 1 gem lettuce broken in a bowl; tossed with 100 g (4½ oz) tuna (in brine, drained); 200 g (7 oz) cooked new potatoes, sliced; tomato; spring onions; watercress; 1 hard-boiled egg (size 3), quartered; 3 black olives; 2 tablespoons reduced-fat French dressing.
  25 g (10 oz) slice of low-fat cheese on a cracker or crispbread.
  125 g (5 oz) low-fat fruit yoghurt.
- Mushroom omelette: a few mushrooms chopped and lightly fried in 1 teaspoon butter plus 1 tablespoon corn oil, add 2 eggs (size 3) whisked with a little skimmed or semi-skimmed milk, seasoning and chopped chives (dried or fresh). Serve with salad with oil-free dressing.
  Slice of wholemeal bread smeared with low-fat spread.
  Fruit from allowance.
- Lamb kebab: 4 x 2.5cm (1 inch) cubes lean lamb; 1 rasher back bacon, well-trimmed and sliced; 1 small onion, quartered; 1 tomato, quartered; ½ green pepper, cut into squares; plus 1 tablespoon barbecue sauce. Serve with 200 g (7 oz) boiled rice or potatoes and green salad from allowance.
  125 g (5 oz) low-fat natural yoghurt.
  Fruit from allowance.
- Pea soup: 100g (4 oz) frozen peas, 50 g (2 oz) chopped onions and 100 g (4 oz) chopped potatoes lightly fried in a non-stick pan with a little oil; add 150 ml (¼ pint) vegetable stock, 150 ml (¼ pint) skimmed milk, and a little dried mint. Bring to the boil and simmer for 15 minutes. Serve with a roll or pitta bread.
  100 g (4 oz) fruit-flavoured fromage frais.

1250
A

- Grilled white fish: medium portion of haddock, cod, or other white fish, grilled or poached, served with 100 g (4 oz) boiled peas, 200 g (7 oz) boiled new potatoes and 1 tablespoon tartare sauce.
25 g (1 oz) slice low-fat cheese on a cracker or crispbread.
Fruit from allowance.
- 100 g (4 oz) pasta, boiled; sauce made from 200 g (7 oz) canned chopped tomatoes (with herbs if preferred), cooked in a little oil and seasoned with ½ teaspoon of sugar and black pepper. Green salad from allowance. 125 g (5 oz) low-fat natural yoghurt.
1 apple, orange, pear, peach.
- 1 skinned medium chicken breast, sliced into small cubes, stir-fried with beansprouts, mushrooms, mangetout or runner beans, herbs and spices to taste. Serve with 200 g (7 oz) boiled rice.
1 medium-sized banana.
- Cauliflower cheese: 175 g (6 oz) cauliflower florets, boiled, covered with a cheese sauce made with 50 g (2 oz) reduced-fat Cheddar, 1 tablespoon cornflour and 175 ml (6 fl oz) skimmed milk. Grilled in an ovenproof dish until bubbling. Green salad from allowance. 125 g (5 oz) low-fat natural yoghurt with 4 ready-to-eat dried apricots or 1 small apple.
- 200 g (7 oz) jacket-baked potato, filled with 150 g (5 oz) baked beans. Salad from allowance.
25 g (1 oz) slice reduced fat cheese on a cracker or crispbread.
1 apple, pear, orange or peach.
- 100 g (4 oz) cooked weight cold pasta shells mixed with 1 medium apple, chopped, and 50 g (2 oz) tuna (in brine, drained) and ½ red pepper, chopped; all tossed in 1 tablespoon reduced-fat French dressing.
25 g (1 oz) slice reduced-fat cheese on a cracker or crispbread.
125 g (5 oz) low-fat fruit yoghurt.
- 300ml (½ pint) canned thick vegetable soup sprinkled with 1 tablespoon grated Parmesan or Cheddar plus 1 crusty roll.
125 g (5 oz) low-fat natural yoghurt. 1 apple, pear, orange, peach.

1250
A

Phase A Snacks/Treats
NONE – Sorry! – but don't forget your 100 calorie fruit allowance (pick from Healthy Xtras 100 list on page 65) and free mixed salad from Ad Lib list also on page 65.

Plan 1250 – PHASE B *(averaging about 1250 cals/day)*

After the austerity of Phase A, things ease up a little in this 'B' for 'Better' phase. You get a bigger breakfast (200 calories), a bigger light meal (300 calories) and an extra 100 calories-worth of treats a day in addition to the usual allowances and ad libs.

Phase B Breakfasts *(about 200 calories)*
Make sure you don't skip breakfast – it is not much but it helps you through the morning. Each day, pick any ONE of the following. Vary your choice from day to day:

- ½ fresh grapefruit; 1 medium slice wholemeal toast with thin smear of low-fat spread.
- 150 ml (¼ pint) unsweetened fruit juice; 40 g (1½ oz) unsweetened muesli; 150 ml (¼ pint) skimmed milk.
- 150 ml (¼ pint) unsweetened fruit juice; 100 g (4 oz) low-fat fromage frais with fruit (or fresh apple/pear chopped in).
- 1 boiled/poached egg (size 3); 1 medium slice wholemeal toast with low-fat spread.
- 1 medium-sized banana; 2 wheat crackers thinly spread with light soft cheese.
- 125 g (5 oz) low-fat natural yoghurt with 25 g (1oz) dried apricots or 1 fresh apple/pear chopped in.
- 1 shredded wheat; 150 ml (¼ pint) skimmed milk; ½ medium-sized banana chopped in.
- 150 ml (¼ pint) unsweetened fruit juice; 1wholewheat bisk; 150 ml (¼ pint) skimmed milk; 2 ready-to-eat dried apricots.
- 125 g (5oz) low-fat natural yoghurt; 1 medium slice wholemeal toast; 2 teaspoons marmalade (without spread).
- 40 g (1½oz) branflakes; 150ml (¼ pint) skimmed milk; topped with 225 g (8 oz) melon or grapefruit segments.

1250
B

Phase B Light Meals *(about 300 calories)*
Each day, pick any ONE of the following. Vary your choice from day to day:

- 200 g (7 oz) jacket-baked potato, filled with 40 g (1½ oz) reduced-fat Cheddar and ½ small onion sliced or chopped in; 1 orange/apple/pear.
- 2 medium slices wholemeal bread; smear of low-fat spread; 25 g (1 oz) lean ham; 1 sliced tomato; 1 orange/apple.
- 1 slimmer's cup-a-soup with 50 g (2 oz) wholemeal bread soft roll; 125 g (5 oz) low-fat fruit yoghurt (any flavour).
- 1 medium avocado filled with 50 g (2 oz) cottage cheese; 1 orange/apple/pear.
- 2 medium slices wholemeal bread; 2 tablespoons light coleslaw; 1 slice well-grilled lean back bacon chopped into filling; lettuce and tomato garnish; 100 g (4 oz) low-fat fromage frais (any flavour).
- 1 rye crispbread; top with 1 hard-boiled egg (size 3) finely diced with low-fat mayonnaise; garnish with capers or sliced tomato; 1 orange/apple/pear.
- 200 g (7 oz) jacket-baked potato; opened and mashed with ½ tablespoon low-fat spread; filled with 150 g (5½ oz) low-sugar baked beans; 1 orange/apple/pear.
- 2 medium slices wholemeal bread; 50 g (2 oz) sardines (drained of oil); unlimited cucumber slices; 125 g (5 oz) low-fat yoghurt (any flavour).
- 1 large wholemeal bap; low-fat spread; lettuce, cucumber and tomato; sliced hard-boiled egg (size 3); low-fat mayonnaise; 100 g (4 oz) low-fat fromage frais (any flavour).
- 200 g (7 oz) jacket-baked potato; filled with 50 g (2 oz) chopped ham and 50g (2oz) diced mushrooms poached in a little skimmed milk; 1 orange/apple/pear.
- 25 g (1 oz) Mozzarella sliced with 1 tomato sliced, garnished with 4 black olives sliced, and 1 small spring onion sliced; sprinkled with ½ tablespoon standard French dressing; plus 75 g (3 oz) slice of long French loaf.
- 2 medium slices wholemeal bread; 50 g (2 oz) liver sausage; unlimited crisp lettuce; unlimited sliced tomato; 1 apple or pear to follow.

1250
B

- Tuna and egg salad made from 1 gem lettuce broken in a bowl; tossed with 100 g (4 oz) tuna (in brine, drained); 200 g (7 oz) cooked new potato, sliced; tomato; spring onions; watercress; 1 hard-boiled egg (size 3), quartered; 3 black olives; 2 tablespoons reduced-fat French dressing.

Phase B Main Meals *(about 450 calories)*
Choose from the Phase A selection beginning on page 83.

Phase B Snacks/Treats *(about 100 calories)*
Preferably something fruity or starchy from the Healthy Xtras 100 list on page 65. But you can choose from the Wicked Treats 100 list if you wish.

- Mix and match as you like, but remember the sensible limit for alcohol (see page 64).
- These extras are in addition to your usual allowances and ad libs (see page 65).

1250
C

Plan 1250 – PHASE C *(averaging about 1750 cals/day)*

This is the 'C' for 'Craving' phase, and, as you can see, it allows three snacks or treats of your choice each day (up to 600 calories-worth) in addition to the three meals and usual allowances. You can use these snacks to help you through the cravings by choosing sugary, starchy or chocolatey things if you like – as long as you keep to the limit.
Remember that the fewer days you spend in this phase of the plan, the faster will be your weight loss.

Phase C Breakfasts *(about 200 calories)*
Choose from the Phase B selection beginning on page 87.

Phase C Light Meals *(about 300 calories)*
Choose from the Phase B selection beginning on page 88.

Phase C Main Meals *(about 450 calories)*
Choose a main meal from either Plan 1250 Phase A selection beginning on page 83 or from the following:
- *Tuna and Vegetable Lasagne* (see page 128) 1 serving;
  Fruit from allowance.
- *Two Cheese Flan* (see page 109) Ⓥ 1 serving;
  1 small banana
- *Italian Rice Chicken* (see page 114) 1 serving;
  150 g (5½ oz) low-fat natural yoghurt and fruit from allowance.

Phase C Snacks/Treats *(about 600 calories in total)*
Select TWO items from the Healthy Xtras 250 list on page 67 (or the Wicked Treats 250 list on page 68 if you wish), plus ONE item from the Healthy Xtras 100 list on page 66 (or the Wicked Treats 100 list on page 00 if you wish).
- Preferably choose starchy things to ease the cravings – but of course the choice is yours.
- Mix and match as you like – but keep to the limit for each item and remember the sensible limits for alcohol (see page 64).
- Use your answers to Question 9 of the 'Know Your Own Body-clock' quiz on page 47 to help decide what time of day to have your starchy snacks.
- You may prefer to bolster your meals with extras or space your snacks evenly throughout the day so that you never have too long to wait.
- These extras are in addition to your usual allowances and ad libs (see page 65).

chapter 9

Body-clock Plan 1500

About this plan

This Body-clock Diet plan provides about 1500 calories a day, averaged over a typical menstrual cycle. This is the plan to follow if you have more than 3 stone to lose in order to reach your target weight. The reason why slimmers who have more to lose are allowed more calories is explained on page 53.

Plan 1500 is designed to be a longer term diet – satisfying, with plenty of variety and delicious recipes. Most women in the above category who start their slimming with this plan can expect to lose up to 5lb in the first week, slightly less in the second week, and 1-2lbs a week after that. So, hopefully, you should reach your target from the sixth cycle onwards, depending on exactly how much you want to lose. But remember, a few of those lost pounds may be 'phantom' ones – in other words water (see page 12).

Menu options

For the main meals, each phase of the plan offers not only a choice of different set menus and recipes – '*Cook's Choice*'– but also, in case you're too short of time or don't want to fiddle about too much, suggestions for something easier and simpler – '*No Fuss*'.

As well as this choice, each phase of the plan also indicates the vegetarian options (marked Ⓥ).

But remember, it's most important that you select only menu options from whichever phase of the plan you are currently going through. Never 'mix' phases.

Here we go...

Plan 1500 – Step by step

1 Before you start, make sure you're familiar with the BASIC STEPS outlined on pages 54-61 and the DIET RULES on pages 63-65.

2 Start the plan at the beginning of your Phase A. Remember that this is the most slimming phase – only 1250 calories a day – so don't delay starting for too long otherwise you may not be able to cover your full 14 days before you find you need to switch to the more calorific Phase B.

3 Don't forget that, if you're following the Body-clock Exercise Programme (see Chapter 11), you can add a 250 calorie extra for every 30 minutes of moderately vigorous activity – such as aerobics, skipping, running or swimming lengths. For example, the High Intensity programme allows you an extra 250 calories-worth a day. Select any item from the Healthy Xtras 250 list on page 67.

4 It's best to switch to Phase B after about fourteen days. Continuing Phase A much beyond that may trigger the 'famine response' (see page 13).

5 Phase B gives you 1500 calories a day and the longer you can stay in it before switching to Phase C the better. You are allowed 250 calories-worth of extras or treats, preferably from the Healthy Xtras 250 list. Phase B may last right up to your next period. But if you get severe cravings, you may have to switch to Phase C.

6 Phase C, usually the last few days of the cycle, is different in several ways. It gives you:
   - more food (increased to about 2000 calories a day)
   - more often (six meals/snacks a day)
   - more carbohydrate to beat the cravings

Because of the more generous calorie allowance during this phase, you should only switch to it if you feel the need – otherwise you will slow down your weight loss unnecessarily.

7 Once you have reached your target, the guidelines in Chapter 12 will help you adjust your calorie intakes to maintain your new slim weight.

Plan 1500 Menus

Make sure you select only from the choices specified for each phase of the plan.

Plan 1500 – PHASE A *(averaging about 1250 cals/day)*

Each day:
- 🍎 select one breakfast, one light meal and one main meal;
- 🍎 plus 'milk' from allowance (see page 65);
- 🍎 plus 100 calories-worth of fruit from Healthy Xtras 100 list (see page 65)
- 🍎 plus Ad Lib salad (see page 65)

Phase A Breakfasts *(about 200 calories)*
Make sure you don't skip breakfast – it's not much but it helps you through the morning. Each day, pick any ONE of the following. Vary your choice from day to day:

- ½ fresh grapefruit; 1 medium slice wholemeal toast with thin smear of low-fat spread, 2 teaspoons jam or marmalade.
- 150 ml (¼ pint) unsweetened fruit juice; 40 g (1½ oz) unsweetened muesli; 150 ml (¼ pint) skimmed milk
- 150 ml (¼ pint) unsweetened fruit juice; 100 g (4 oz) low-fat fromage frais with fruit (or fresh apple/pear chopped in).
- 1 boiled/poached egg (size 3); 1 medium slice wholemeal toast with low-fat spread.
- 1 medium-sized banana; 2 wheat crackers thinly spread with light soft cheese.
- 150 ml (¼ pint) unsweetened fruit juice; 125 g (5 oz) low-fat natural yoghurt with 25 g (1 oz) dried apricots or fresh apple/pear chopped in.
- 1 shredded wheat; 150 ml (¼ pint) skimmed milk; ½ medium-sized banana chopped in.
- 150 ml (¼ pint) unsweetened fruit juice; 1 wholewheat bisk; 150 ml (¼ pint) skimmed milk; 2 ready-to-eat dried apricots.

1500
A

- 125 g (5 oz) low-fat natural yoghurt; 1 medium slice wholemeal toast; 2 teaspoons marmalade (without spread).
- 40 g (1½ oz) branflakes; 150 ml (¼ pint) skimmed milk; topped with 225g (8 oz) melon or grapefruit segments.
- 125 g (5 oz) low-fat natural yoghurt plus 1 medium banana.
- 150 ml (¼ pint) unsweetened fruit juice; 25 g (1oz) cornflakes; 150 ml (¼ pint) skimmed milk.
- Fruit salad made with 1 orange, 1 apple, a few seedless grapes, 1 small banana, 4 tablespoons unsweetened orange juice.
- 1 English muffin, toasted, smear of low-fat spread, smear of honey.

Phase A Light Meals *(about 300 calories)*
Each day, pick any ONE of the following. Vary your choice from day to day:
- 200 g (7 oz) jacket-baked potato, filled with 40 g (1½ oz) reduced-fat Cheddar and ½ small onion sliced or chopped in; 1 orange/apple/pear.
- 2 medium slices wholemeal bread; smear of low-fat spread; 25 g (1 oz) lean ham; 1 sliced tomato; 1 orange/apple.
- 1 slimmer's cup-a-soup with 50g (2oz) wholemeal bread soft roll; 125g (5oz) low-fat fruit yoghurt (any flavour).
- 1 medium avocado filled with 50 g (2 oz) cottage cheese; 1 orange/apple/pear.
- 2 medium slices wholemeal bread; 2 tablespoons light coleslaw; 1 slice well-grilled lean back bacon chopped into filling; lettuce and tomato garnish; 100 g (4 oz) low-fat fromage frais (any flavour).
- 1 rye crispbread; topped with 1 hard-boiled egg (size 3) finely diced with low-fat mayonnaise; garnished with capers or sliced tomato; 1 orange/apple/pear.
- 200 g (7 oz) jacket-baked potato; opened and mashed with ½ a tablespoon low-fat spread; filled with 150 g (5½oz) low-sugar baked beans; 1 orange/apple/pear.
- 2 medium slices wholemeal bread; 50 g (2 oz) sardines (drained of oil); unlimited cucumber slices; 125 g (5 oz) low-fat yoghurt (any flavour).

1500
A

- 1 large wholemeal bap; smear of low-fat spread; lettuce, cucumber and tomato;1 sliced hard-boiled egg (size 3); low-fat mayonnaise; 100 g (4 oz) low-fat fromage frais (any flavour).
- 200g (7oz) jacket-baked potato; filled with 50 g (2 oz) chopped ham and 50g (2oz) diced mushrooms poached in a little skimmed milk; 1 orange/apple/pear.
- 25 g (1 oz) Mozzarella sliced with 1 tomato sliced, garnished with 4 black olives sliced, and 1 small spring onion sliced; sprinkled with ½ tablespoon standard French dressing; plus 75 g (3 oz) slice of long French loaf.
- 2 medium slices wholemeal bread; 50 g (2 oz) liver sausage; unlimited crisp lettuce; unlimited sliced tomato; 1 apple or pear to follow.
- Tuna and egg salad made from 1 gem lettuce broken in a bowl; tossed with 100 g (4 oz) tuna (in brine, drained); 200 g (7 oz) cooked new potato, sliced; tomato; spring onions; watercress; 1 hard-boiled egg (size 3), quartered; 3 black olives; 2 tablespoons reduced-fat French dressing.

Phase A Main Meals *(about 550 calories)*
Each day, pick any ONE complete meal from either the 'Cooks' Choice' or 'No Fuss' lists (preferably something quite different from your light meal). Vary your choice from day to day.

1500
A

'Cooks' Choice' Menus
- *Tuna and Egg Salad* (see page 123) 1 serving;
  Summer Pudding (see page129) 1 serving.
- *Turkey Two-Pepper Salad* (see page 111) 1 serving;
  Strawberry Parfait (see page130) 1 serving.
- *Gammon and Spicy Pineapple* (see page 111) 1 serving;
  Potatoes and vegetables;
  100 g (4 oz) low-fat fromage frais.
- *Devilled Kidneys* (see page 113) 1 serving;
  Winter Fruit Flan (see page131) 1 serving.

- *Spicy Bean Hot Pot* (see page 107) Ⓥ 1 serving;
  Crunchy Nectarines (see page 131) 1 serving.
- *Cod, Leek and Potato Bake* (see page126) 1 serving;
  Spicy Compote (see page 133) 1 serving.
- *Fish Curry* (see page 127) 1 serving;
  Lemon Sponge Pudding (see page 132) 1 serving.
- *Baked Chicken and Peppers* (see page 117) 1 serving;
  Jacket-baked potato and green salad;
  Crunchy Nectarines (see page 131).
- *Ham and Prawn Jambalaya* (see page 113) 1 serving;
  125 g (5 oz) low-fat fruit yoghurt.
- *Spaghetti Bolognese* (see page 117);
  125 g (5 oz) low-fat natural yoghurt;
  Fruit from allowance.
- *Apricot Lamb Pilaf* (see page 119) 1 serving;
  25 g (1oz) reduced-fat cheese and a cracker;
  100 g (4 oz) low-fat fruit fromage frais.
- *Fish with Peppers* (see page122) 1 serving;
  2-3 small new potatoes, plus;
  125 g (5 oz) low-fat natural yoghurt and 2 semi-dried apricots.
- *Prawn and Mushroom Risotto* (see page 123) 1 serving;
  Strawberry Parfait (see page 130).
- *Pasta Stroganoff* (see page 105) Ⓥ 1 serving;
  Spicy Compote (see page 133).
- *Tuna Tagliatelle* (see page 125) 1 serving;
  Green salad from allowance;
  Fruity Fool (see page 133), 1 serving.
- *Liver and Bacon Casserole* (see page 115) 1 serving;
  Spicy Compote (see page 133), 1 serving.
- *Eggs Florentine* (see page 107) Ⓥ 1 serving;
  125 g (5 oz) low-fat natural yoghurt;
  1 apple, pear, orange or nectarine.

1500
A

'No Fuss' Menus (about 550 calories)
NOTE: Each of the following serves ONE slimmer only. Multiply quantities by four to serve two children and one non-slimming adult as well as yourself.

- 100 g (4 oz) gammon rasher, grilled; plus 200 g (7 oz) jacket-baked potato filled with 25 g (1 oz) cottage cheese; plus 25 g (1 oz) frozen peas, boiled. 1 slice reduced-fat cheese on a cracker or crispbread. 125 g (5 oz) low-fat natural yoghurt and fruit from allowance.

- 1 thick slice wholemeal toast,150 g (5½ oz) baked beans, 2 low-fat chipolata sausages and 1 poached egg (size 3). 125 g (5 oz) low-fat natural yoghurt 1 apple, pear, orange.

- 100 g (4 oz) well-trimmed chump lamb or pork chop, grilled; 100 g (4 oz) potato, boiled; 100g (4oz) frozen broccoli or other vegetable, steamed or boiled. 25 g (1 oz) slice reduced-fat cheese on a cracker or crispbread. 1 portion fruit salad (in juice) and 1 tbsp half-fat cream.

- Tuna and egg salad:1 gem lettuce; tossed with 100 g (4 oz) tuna (in brine, drained); 200 g (7 oz) cooked new potato, sliced; tomato; spring onions; watercress; 1 hard-boiled egg (size 3), quartered; 3 black olives; 2 tablespoons reduced-fat French dressing. 1 wholemeal roll and 1 tablespoon low-fat spread. 1 medium banana.

- Mushroom omelette: a few mushrooms chopped and lightly fried in 1 teaspoon butter plus 1 tablespoon corn oil, add 2 eggs (size 3) whisked with a little skimmed or semi-skimmed milk, seasoning and chopped chives (dried or fresh). Serve with wholemeal roll and salad with oil-free dressing. 125 g (5 oz) low-fat fruit yoghurt.

- Lamb kebab: grill 4 x 2.5 cm (1inch) cubes lean lamb; 1 rasher back bacon, trimmed and sliced; 1 small onion, quartered; 1 tomato, quartered; ½ green pepper, cut into squares; plus 1 tbsp barbecue sauce. Serve with 200 g (7 oz) boiled rice or potatoes and green salad from allowance. 25 g (1 oz) slice reduced-fat cheese on a cracker or crispbread. Fruit salad in juice plus 1 tbsp half cream.

- Pea soup: 100 g (4 oz) frozen peas, 50 g (2 oz) chopped onions and 100 g (4 oz) chopped potatoes lightly fried in a non-stick pan with a little oil; add 150 ml (¼ pint) vegetable stock, 150 ml (¼ pint) skimmed milk, and a little dried mint. Bring to the boil and simmer for 15 minutes. Serve with a roll or pitta bread. 120 g (4½oz) frozen fruit fool.

1500
A

- Medium portion of haddock, cod, or other white fish, grilled or poached, served with 100 g (4 oz) peas, 200 g (7 oz) boiled new potatoes and 1 tablespoon tartare sauce. 25 g (1 oz) slice reduced-fat cheese on a cracker or crispbread. 1 medium banana.
- 100 g (4 oz) pasta, boiled; plus a sauce made from 200 g (7 oz) canned chopped tomatoes (with herbs if preferred), cooked in a little oil and seasoned with ½ teaspoon of sugar and black pepper. Serve with a green salad from allowance. 25 g (1 oz) slice reduced-fat cheese on a cracker or crispbread. 125 g (5 oz) low-fat natural yoghurt. 1 apple, orange, pear or nectarine.
- 1 skinned medium chicken breast, sliced into small cubes, stir-fried with beansprouts, mushrooms, mangetout or runner beans, herbs and spices to taste. Serve with 200 g (7 oz) boiled rice. 1 medium-sized banana.
- 175 g (6 oz) cauliflower florets, boiled, covered with a cheese sauce made with 50 g (2 oz) reduced-fat Cheddar, 1 tablespoon cornflour and 175 ml (6 fl oz) skimmed milk. Grill in an ovenproof dish until bubbling. Green salad from allowance. 1 wholemeal roll. 125 g (5 oz) low-fat natural yoghurt with 4 ready-to-eat dried apricots.
- 200 g (7 oz) jacket-baked potato, filled with 150 g (5½oz) baked beans. Salad from allowance. Slice of low-fat cheese on a cracker or crispbread. 125g (5oz) low-fat natural yoghurt. 1 apple, pear, orange or nectarine.
- 100g (4oz) cooked weight cold pasta shells mixed with 1 medium apple, chopped, 50g (2oz) tuna (in brine, drained) and ½ red pepper, chopped; all tossed in 1 tablespoon reduced-fat French dressing. 25 g (1 oz) slice of reduced-fat cheese on a cracker or crispbread. 100 g (4 oz) frozen chocolate mousse. Fruit from allowance.
- 300 ml (½ pint) canned thick vegetable soup sprinkled with 1 tablespoon grated Parmesan or Cheddar, plus 1 crusty roll. 1 individual fruit pie plus 1 tablespoon half cream.

1500 A

Phase A Snacks/Treats

NONE! – Sorry! – but don't forget your 100-calorie fruit allowance (pick from the Healthy Xtras 100 list on page 65) and free mixed salad from the Ad Lib list also on page 65.

Plan 1500 – PHASE B *(averaging about 1500 cals/day)*

After the austerity of Phase A, things ease up a little in this 'B' for 'Better' phase. You are allowed 250 calories-worth of extra snacks/treats a day in addition to meals, allowances and ad libs!

Phase B Breakfasts *(about 200 calories)*
Choose from the Phase A selection beginning on page 93.

Phase B Light Meals *(about 300 calories)*
Choose from the Phase A selection beginning on page 94.

Phase B Main meals *(about 550 calories)*
Choose from the Phase A selection beginning on page 95.

Phase B Snacks/Treats *(about 250 calories)*
Preferably something fruity or starchy from the Healthy Xtras 250 list on page 67. But you can choose from the Wicked Treats 250 list if you wish.
- Mix and match as you like, but remember the sensible limit for alcohol (see page 64).
- These extras are in addition to your usual allowances and ad libs (see page 65)

1500
B

PLAN 1500 – PHASE C *(averaging about 2000 cals/day)*

This is the 'C' for 'Craving' phase, and, as you can see, it allows three snacks or treats of your choice each day (up to 750 calories-worth) in addition to the three meals and ad libs. You can use these snacks to help you through the cravings by choosing starchy, sugary or chocolatey things if you like – as long as you keep to the limit.
Remember that the fewer days you spend in this phase of the plan, the faster will be your weight loss.

Phase C Breakfasts *(about 200 calories)*
Choose from the Phase A selection beginning on page 93.

Phase C Light Meals *(about 300 calories)*
Choose one light meal from the Phase A selection beginning on page 94.

Phase C Main Meals *(about 550 calories)*
Choose from the Phase A selection beginning on page 95.

Phase C Snacks/Treats *(about 750 calories)*
Select THREE items from the Healthy Xtras 250 list on page 67 (or Wicked Treats 250 lists if you wish).

- Preferably choose starchy things to help combat the cravings – but of course the choice is yours.
- Use your answers to Question 9 of the 'Know Your Own Body-clock' quiz on page 47 to help decide when best to have your starchy snacks.
- You may prefer to bolster your meals with extras or space your snacks evenly throughout the day so that you never have too long to wait.
- Mix and match as you like – but keep to the limit for each item and remember the sensible limits for alcohol (see page 64).
- These extras are in addition to your usual allowances and ad libs (see page 65).

1500
C

CHAPTER 10

The Body-clock Diet Recipes

Stuffed Peppers Ⓥ

Serves 4; 200 calories per serving

100 g (4 oz) brown rice
Salt
4 green or red peppers
1 medium onion, finely
    chopped
40 g (1½ oz) sunflower seeds

40 g (1½ oz) dried apricots,
    chopped
½ teaspoon dried thyme or 1
    teaspoon fresh thyme
1 size 3 egg
250 ml (8 fl oz) tomato juice

Simmer the rice in lightly salted boiling water for 20 minutes. Drain. Halve the peppers and de-seed. Mix the onion, sunflower seeds, apricots, thyme and egg with the rice, and stuff the mixture into the peppers. Place, with the tomato juice, in a hot oven and bake for 30-40 minutes.

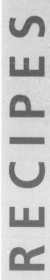
RECIPES

Vegetable Moussaka Ⓥ

Serves 4; 350 calories per serving

2 medium-sized aubergines
2 tablespoons salt
1 tablespoon sunflower oil
225 g (8 oz) mushrooms,
    sliced
2 cloves garlic, crushed
4 sticks of celery, sliced
2 medium leeks, sliced
2 x 400 g (14 oz) cans
    chopped tomatoes

450 ml (¾ pint) semi-skimmed
    milk
3 heaped tablespoons flour
100 g (4 oz) low-fat soft
    cheese
50 g (2 oz) half-fat Cheddar,
    grated

Cut the aubergines into 1cm (½in) slices. Sprinkle with the salt and leave for 30 minutes to absorb the bitter juices. Rinse off the salt with cold water and dab dry. Heat the oil in a pan and gently fry the mushrooms and garlic for 3 minutes. Blanch the celery and leeks iin boiling water for 2 minutes and drain. Drain the tomatoes. Mix 4 tbsp of the milk with the flour to make a smooth paste. Stir in the remaining milk and heat gently in a saucepan until it thickens. Blend in the soft cheese. Spread out half the aubergine slices to cover the base of a large ovenproof dish. Add the mushrooms and garlic mixture, spreading it out. Add half the tomatoes to make another layer. Then a layer of the leeks and celery. Then the rest of the aubergines, and the rest of the tomatoes. Top with the sauce, sprinkled with the grated cheese. Bake in a pre-heated moderate oven 200° C/400° F/Gas 6 until brown (25-30 minutes). Serve with lettuce and black olive salad.

RECIPES

Cheese and Pineapple Pizza Ⓥ

Serves 4; 330 calories per serving

4 tomatoes, peeled and
    chopped
2 cloves garlic, finely chopped
2 medium onions, finely
    chopped
½ teaspoon dried basil or 2
    teaspoons finely chopped
    fresh basil
2 tablespoons tomato paste

2 large wholemeal pitta
    breads, halved (or 4 small
    pizza bases)
125 g (5 oz) unsweetened
    pineapple chunks, crushed
100 g (4 oz) Edam or low-fat
    Cheddar, grated
2 tablespoons Parmesan,
    grated
Black pepper to taste

Mix the tomatoes, garlic, onions, basil and tomato paste in a saucepan and simmer for about 10 minutes. Spread over the pitta bread (or pizza bases). Top with the pineapple and cheese. Bake in a pre-heated hot oven 220°C/425°F/Gas 7 until brown (about 15 minutes). Sprinkle with Parmesan and black pepper and serve.

Red Pepper Pasta Ⓥ

Serves 4; 300 calories per serving

225 g (8 oz) pasta twists
Salt
2 medium-sized red peppers

Sprinkling of fresh or dried
    sage
½ tablespoon French dressing

Add the pasta to boiling slightly salted water, and cook until soft. Drain and cool. Quarter the peppers, removing stalk and seeds. Grill the peppers until skins are blackened. Cool and peel them. Cut them into thin strips and toss them with the pasta, sage and dressing. Serve cold.

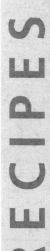

Baked Bean Gratin Ⓥ

Serves 4; 300 calories per serving

8 medium-sized tomatoes,
   sliced
2 x 450 g (1lb) cans baked
   beans in tomato sauce

50 g (2 oz) Edam, grated
100 g (4 oz) breadcrumbs

Spread the tomato slices over the base of a large gratin dish. Heat the beans and spread them over the tomatoes. Mix the cheese and breadcrumbs together and sprinkle over the beans, forming an even layer. Grill until crisp, sizzling and tinged with brown. Serve hot.

Spiced Chick Peas Ⓥ

Serves 4; 250 calories per serving

1 tablespoon sunflower oil
1 large onion, chopped
1 teaspoon turmeric
1 teaspoon cumin
2 green chillies, de-seeded
   and chopped
2 x 400 g (14 oz) cans
   cooked chick peas,
   drained

2 x 400 g (14 oz) cans
   chopped tomatoes
1 tablespoon lemon juice
Black pepper to taste
3 tablespoons fresh coriander,
   chopped

Heat the oil in a saucepan and gently fry the onion until soft. Add the turmeric, cumin and chillies, and stir-fry for 2-3 minutes. Add the chick peas, tomatoes, lemon juice and season with freshly ground black pepper. Stir-fry for a further 3-4 minutes. Serve sprinkled with the coriander.

RECIPES

Pasta Stroganoff Ⓥ

Serves 4; 400 calories per serving

225 g (8 oz) dry pasta
1 teaspoon olive oil
1 medium onion, finely
   chopped
100 g (4 oz) mushrooms,
   sliced

2 tablespoons white wine
1 teaspoon fresh marjoram
65 g (2½ oz) low-fat natural
   yoghurt
Black pepper to taste
3 tablespoons Parmesan

Cook the pasta in boiling lightly salted water and drain.Heat the oil in a saucepan and gently fry the onion until soft. Add the mushrooms, wine and marjoram. Cover and simmer for about 10 minutes. Stir in the yoghurt, season with freshly ground pepper, and pour on to the pasta, mixing well. Serve with a sprinkling of Parmesan.

Leek and Potato Soup Ⓥ

Serves 4; 150 calories per serving

15 g (½ oz) butter or
   margarine
1 small onion, peeled and
   chopped
450 g (1 lb) leeks, trimmed
   and chopped

225 g (8 oz) potatoes, peeled
   and diced
900 ml (1½ pints) water or
   vegetable or chicken stock
Salt and black pepper to taste
150 ml (¼ pint) skimmed milk

Melt the butter in a saucepan and fry the onion gently until brown. Add the leeks and potatoes and fry for another 3-5 minutes. Add the stock and seasoning, bring to the boil and simmer until the potatoes are soft (about 30 minutes). Purée the mixture in a blender until smooth. Return the mixture to the saucepan, add the skimmed milk, and re-heat. Serve hot with a garnish of sprinkled, chopped fresh parsley or grated cheese.

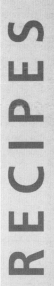

Eggs Florentine Ⓥ

Serves 4; 400 calories per serving

8 eggs (size 3)
675 g (1½ lb) frozen spinach
Black pepper
Large pinch of ground
    nutmeg
50 g (2 oz) low-fat spread

2 heaped tablespoons plain
    flour
450 ml (¾ pint) skimmed milk
100 g (4 oz) reduced-fat hard
    cheese, grated

Hard boil the eggs. Meanwhile, steam the spinach and thoroughly drain it. Season with pepper and nutmeg and place in an ovenproof dish. Slice the eggs and arrange on top of the spinach. Mix the low-fat spread, flour and skimmed milk in a pan, bring to the boil and whisk until thickened. Stir in the grated cheese and pour over the eggs. Grill until cheese sauce bubbles.

Spicy Bean Hot Pot Ⓥ

Serves 4; 400 calories per serving

2 medium onions, chopped
2 celery sticks, sliced
1 tablespoon sunflower or
    corn oil
4 cloves garlic, crushed
1 teaspoon chilli powder
1 teaspoon ground coriander
½ teaspoon ground ginger
300 g (11 oz) new potatoes,
    scrubbed and sliced
2 x 400 g (14 oz) cans
    chopped tomatoes

2 x 425 g (15 oz) cans butter
    beans
2 x 225 g (8 oz) cans
    reduced-sugar baked
    beans
200 g (7 oz) broad beans
150 ml (¼ pint) water
Salt and black pepper to taste
200 g (7 oz) cooked weight
    brown rice

Gently fry the onions and celery in the oil for about 5 minutes. Stir in the garlic and spices for a further minute. Add the potatoes and tomatoes, bring to the boil and cook for about 10 minutes. Add the beans and water, bring to the boil and simmer for a further 10 minutes, stirring continuously. Season to taste, add the rice and heat through and then serve.

Satay Salad Ⓥ

Serves 4; 250 calories per serving

100 g (4 oz) brown rice
75 g (3 oz) mangetout
75 g (3 oz) carrots, peeled and grated
100 g (4 oz) cherry tomatoes, halved
50 g (2 oz) radishes, sliced
6 spring onions, chopped
75 g (3 oz) canned baby corn, drained
450 g (1lb) can pineapple chunks in juice

2 teaspoons sesame oil
1 teaspoon white wine vinegar
1 tablespoon fresh coriander, finely chopped (optional)
Rind of 1 lemon, grated
1 clove garlic, crushed
Black pepper to taste
15 g (½ oz) roasted peanuts, peeled and crushed

Cook the rice in lightly salted water, drain and rinse in cold water to cool. Cook the mangetout in boiling water for 1-2 minutes, drain and cool. Toss the rice, mangetout, carrots, tomatoes, radishes, spring onions and sweetcorn together in a salad bowl. Drain the pineapple, reserving the juice. Toss the pineapple into the salad. In a screw-top jar, shake the pineapple juice, oil, vinegar, coriander, lemon rind, garlic and freshly ground black pepper, for 1-2 minutes. Pour the dressing over the salad, garnish with the crushed peanuts and serve.

RECIPES

Two Cheese Flan Ⓥ

Serves 4; 380 calories per serving

175 g (6 oz) plain flour
75 g (3 oz) low-fat spread
1 tablespoon Cheddar
   cheese, grated
175 g (6 oz) baby courgettes
1 teaspoon oil
75 g (3 oz) cherry tomatoes

2 eggs (size 3)
200 ml (7 fl oz) semi-
   skimmed milk
Black pepper to taste
75 g (3 oz) blue cheese such
   as Stilton

Pre-heat the oven to 200° C/400° F/Gas 6. Put the flour in a mixing bowl and rub in the low-fat spread. Sprinkle in the grated Cheddar and enough cold water to make a dough with cheesy lumps. Roll out and lay on a medium-sized, lightly greased flan tin. Bake for 10 minutes. Meanwhile, trim and slice the courgettes lengthways. Heat the oil in a pan and gently fry the courgettes for a few minutes to soften them. Halve the cherry tomatoes and arrange them, with the courgettes, on the flan case. Beat the eggs with the milk and black pepper in the mixing bowl. Pour the mixture over the vegetables. Crumble or grate the blue cheese and scatter over the top. Bake for about 30 minutes at 180°C/350° F/Gas 4 until just turning brown.

French Onion Soup

Serves 4; 380 calories per serving

2 tablespoons olive or corn
   oil
1 tablespoon low-fat spread
2 medium onions, finely sliced
2 level tablespoons plain flour
1.2 litres (2 pints) beef stock

125 g (5 oz) French stick
   bread
75 g (3 oz) Gruyère or
   Cheddar, grated
Fresh parsley, chopped, to
   garnish

Heat the oil and low-fat spread in a large pan, until bubbling. Add the onions and gently fry until brown, about 20 minutes. Stir in the flour and cook for a further minute. Remove from the heat and stir in the stock. Return to the heat and bring to the boil. Cover and simmer for 30 minutes. Slice the bread into 2.5 cm (1inch) slices and sprinkle with the cheese. Grill until bubbling. When the soup is ready to serve, float the bread on top and garnish with the parsley.

Sausage and Corn Cheese Muffins

Serves 4; 400 calories per serving

4 low-fat sausages
3 tablespoons tomato purée
3 tablespoons tomato
 ketchup
½ teaspoon dried mixed herbs
Salt and black pepper to taste
4 wholemeal muffins

100 g (4 oz) mushrooms,
 diced
100 g (4 oz) can sweetcorn,
 drained
100 g (4 oz) reduced-fat
 Cheddar, grated

Grill the sausages. Meanwhile, mix the tomato purée, tomato ketchup, herbs and seasoning in a bowl. Cut the muffins in half and toast the outsides. Spread the tomato mixture over the flat sides. Slice the sausages thinly and arrange over the tomato layer. Mix the mushrooms and sweetcorn and place on the sausage. Sprinkle with the Cheddar. Grill for 4-5 minutes until the cheese bubbles.

RECIPES

Turkey Two-Pepper Salad

Serves 4; 350 calories per serving

8 shallots or 4 small onions,
sliced
225 g (8 oz) red pepper,
de-seeded and sliced
225 g (8 oz) yellow pepper,
de-seeded and sliced
225 g (8 oz) can baby
sweetcorn
20 cherry tomatoes, halved
225 g (8 oz) avocado pear,
peeled and chopped
350 g (¾ lb) cooked turkey
breast, diced

½ teaspoon basil or oregano,
fresh chopped or dried, to
garnish

Dressing:
6 tablespoons unsweetened
apple juice
4 teaspoons clear honey
2 teaspoons wholegrain
mustard
Salt and black pepper to taste

Mix the vegetables, avocado and turkey in a large salad bowl. Whisk together the apple juice, honey, mustard and seasoning in a small bowl, and pour over the salad. Toss lightly and serve with sprinkling of basil or oregano, accompanied by a wholemeal roll (not included in calorie count).

Gammon and Spicy Pineapple

Serves 4; 370 calories per serving;
(excluding potatoes and vegetables)

4 x 120 g (4 oz) slices of
gammon, trimmed
100 ml (3½ fl oz)
unsweetened orange juice
1 tablespoon demerara sugar

1 medium-sized orange
225 g (8 oz) can pineapple
chunks in juice
¼ teaspoon ground allspice
2 teaspoons cornflour

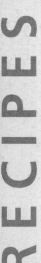

RECIPES

Grill the gammon until done. Meanwhile gently heat the orange juice and sugar in a small pan. Peel, the orange, remove pith and pips and cut into segments. Add to the pan with the pineapple chunks (including juice) and allspice. Cook gently for 2-3 minutes. Blend the cornflour with a little water and add to the pan, stirring until thickened. Cut the gammon into short strips and transfer to the sauce for a few minutes. Serve accompanied by 100 g (4 oz) peas, green beans or broccoli and 100 g (4 oz) small potatoes (adding about 150 calories per serving).

Turkey Stir-Fry

Serves 4; 350 calories per serving

tablespoon corn or
   sunflower oil
2 spring onions, sliced
2 cloves garlic, crushed
2.5 cm (1 inch) piece root
   ginger, grated
1 stick celery, thinly sliced
1 medium-sized onion, diced
350 g (12 oz) turkey breast,
   sliced and chopped
1 green pepper, de-seeded
   and diced

100 g (4 oz) baby sweetcorn
100 g (4 oz) frozen peas or
   broccoli florets
2 tablespoons soy sauce
1 tablespoon sherry
1 teaspoon chilli sauce
1 pinch Chinese 5-spice
4 tablespoons stock
1 tablespoon lemon juice
225 g (8 oz) instant egg
   noodles

Heat the oil in a wok or large frying pan. Gently fry the spring onions, garlic and ginger until soft. Add the celery, onion and turkey. Stir-fry over a high heat for about 3 minutes. Add the remaining vegetables and stir for another 3 minutes. Mix the soy sauce, sherry, chilli sauce, spice, stock and lemon juice and stir into the wok. Bring to the boil. Cook the egg noodles in lightly salted water, and serve with the stir-fry.

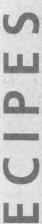

RECIPES

RECIPES

Devilled Kidneys

Serves 4; 270 calories per serving (excluding potatoes)

675 g (1½) lambs' kidneys
25 g (1 oz) plain flour
¼ teaspoon oregano
Salt and black pepper to taste
2 tablespoons oil
2 small onions, chopped

2 green peppers, de-seeded
   and sliced
300 ml (½ pint) lamb, chicken
   or vegetable stock
2 teaspoons English mustard
2 teaspoons Worcester sauce

Remove skin from kidneys, slice lengthways, remove white core. Put the flour in a bowl, mix in the oregano and season with salt and black pepper. Turn the kidneys in the flour mixture. Heat the oil in a pan and lightly fry the onions for 1-2 minutes. Add the kidneys and green peppers and stir-fry until slightly brown. Stir in any remaining flour, the stock, mustard and Worcester sauce. Bring to the boil, cover and simmer for 15-20 minutes. Serve with boiled or baked potatoes

Ham and Prawn Jambalaya

Serves 4; 450 calories per serving

2 tablespoons sunflower oil
1 medium-sized green
   pepper, de-seeded and
   sliced
1 medium-sized onion, diced
2 cloves garlic, crushed
100 g (4 oz) diced lean ham
225 g (8 oz) shelled prawns,
   fresh or frozen

2 x 400 g (14 oz) cans
   tomatoes
1 teaspoon mixed herbs
150 ml (¼ pint) dry white
   wine
225 g (8 oz) long-grain rice

Heat the oil in a flameproof casserole and stir-fry the pepper, onion and garlic until soft. Add the ham and prawns and stir-fry for a few more minutes. Add the tomatoes, herbs and wine, and stir well. Add the rice, bring to the boil, cover and simmer for 30 minutes, stirring frequently.

Italian Rice Chicken

Serves 4, 350 calories per serving

1 tablespoon olive oil
200 g (7 oz) risotto or long-
    grain rice
1 medium onion, chopped
180 g (6 oz) mushrooms,
    sliced
1 red pepper, de-seeded and
    diced
1 green pepper, de-seeded
    and diced

900 ml (1½ pints) chicken
    stock
350 g (12 oz) cooked chicken
    breasts, skinned, boned
    and cut into chunks
1½ teaspoons dried oregano
Salt and black pepper to taste
4 teaspoons grated Parmesan
    to serve

Heat the oil in a large pan and gently fry the rice for a few minutes without browning. Add the onion, mushrooms and peppers and cook for a further 5 minutes. Pour in the stock, cover and simmer over a low heat for about 20 minutes, stirring frequently and adding extra water if necessary. Add the chicken and oregano, turn up the heat and cook for a few minutes. Season with salt and black pepper to taste and serve, sprinkled with the Parmesan.

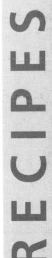

RECIPES

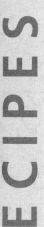

Bacon and Potato Bake

Serves 4; 380 calories per serving

675 g (1½ lb) peeled potatoes
1 egg (size 3)
50 g (2 oz) low-fat spread
225 g (8 oz) lean back bacon
200 g (7 oz) can sweetcorn,
   drained

225 g (8 oz) cottage cheese
   with chives
Salt and black pepper to taste
Chopped fresh chives, to
   garnish

Boil the potatoes until soft, and drain off the water. Beat the egg in a cup and add to the potatoes with the low-fat spread. Mash with a fork until creamy. Grill the bacon and cut or break into small pieces. Stir the sweetcorn and cottage cheese into the mash, mixing thoroughly. Add salt and pepper to taste. Spread the mixture into a large ovenproof dish. Place in a pre-heated hot oven 220°C/425°F/Gas 7 and bake until it begins to brown (25-30 minutes). Sprinkle with chopped chives and serve with a green salad.

Liver and Bacon Casserole

Serves 4; 390 calories per serving

2 x 25 g (1 oz) rashers streaky
   bacon
450 g (1lb) lambs' liver, sliced
400 g (14 oz) can chopped
   tomatoes

1 teaspoon dried thyme
4 tablespoons water
675 g (1½lb) potatoes, peeled
   and sliced
2 teaspoons oil

Grill the bacon and dice. Put it in a casserole dish together with the liver, tomatoes, thyme and water. Cover with the potatoes as a layer. Brush these with the oil, cover and cook in an oven pre-heated to 190°C/375°F/Gas 5 for about 45 minutes. Remove the lid and cook for about 20 minutes more to brown the potatoes.

Sausage Hotpot

Serves 4; 350 calories per serving

450 g (1 lb) new potatoes
8 reduced-fat chipolatas
2 teaspoons cornflour
150 ml (¼ pint) dry cider or
    water

1 tablespoon tomato purée
675 g (1½ lb) canned baked
    beans
Chopped fresh parsley

Boil the potatoes until soft, drain and cut in half. Grill the sausages well, slice into chunks. Put the potatoes and sausages in a large casserole dish. Mix the cornflour with the cider or water making a smooth paste. Pour this mixture into a saucepan, add the tomato purée and bring to the boil, stirring continuously. Add the baked beans to the mixture and stir gently. Pour the mixture over the potatoes and sausages, cover and cook for 15-20 minutes in a pre-heated hot oven 220° C/425° F/Gas 7. Sprinkle with parsley and serve with green salad.

Chilli con Carne

Serves 4; 350 calories per serving

450 g (1 lb) lean minced beef
1 large onion, chopped
1 red pepper, de-seeded and
    chopped
400 g (14 oz) can chopped
    tomatoes

2 tablespoons tomato purée
400 g (14 oz) can red kidney
    beans, drained
2 teaspoons chilli powder
Salt and black pepper to taste

Dry-fry the beef in a non-stick pan until brown and remove from the pan. Add the onion and cook for about 5 minutes. Add the pepper and cook for 5 more minutes. Return the mince with the tomatoes, tomato purée, beans and chilli. Mix well and bring to the boil. Cover and simmer for about 30 minutes, stirring occasionally. Season to taste.

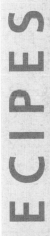

RECIPES

Spaghetti Bolognese

Serves 4; 450 calories per serving

1 tablespoon olive or
  sunflower oil
2 medium onions, finely
  chopped
3 cloves garlic, sliced
2 sticks celery, sliced
2 medium carrots, grated

450 g (1 lb) lean minced beef
400 g (14 oz) can tomatoes
2 tablespoons tomato purée
Pinch dried oregano
200 g (7 oz) spaghetti
Black pepper to taste

Heat the oil in a pan and gently fry the onions, garlic and celery until softened. Add the carrots and mince and stir-cook until the mince is brown. Add the tomatoes, tomato purée and oregano. Bring to the boil, cover and simmer for 30 minutes. Meanwhile, cook the spaghetti in boiling lightly salted water for 10-12 minutes. Drain and serve topped with the bolognese sauce. Season with black pepper to taste

Baked Chicken and Peppers

Serves 4; 250 calories per serving; (excluding jacket-baked potato 150 calories)

2 tablespoons oil
1 medium onion, sliced
1 red pepper, de-seeded and
  sliced
1 yellow pepper, de-seeded
  and sliced

2 tablespoons breadcrumbs
Salt and black pepper to taste
4 x 100 g (4 oz) chicken
  breasts, meat only
300 ml (½ pint) chicken stock

RECIPES

Heat half of the oil in a flameproof casserole and gently cook the onion for about 5 minutes. Add the peppers and cook for 5 more minutes, stirring occasionally. Remove from the heat. Put the remaining oil in a cup and stir in the breadcrumbs and seasoning (including paprika if you wish). Brush this mixture over the chicken breasts, and place the chicken on top of the onions and peppers. Pour in the chicken stock. Cover and bake for about 45 minutes in an oven preheated to 190°C/375°F/Gas 5. Serve with 200 g (7 oz) jacket-baked potato and green salad from allowance.

Lamb and Potato Fry

Serves 4; 290 calories per serving

1 aubergine, thinly sliced
Salt
2 tablespoons oil
450 g (1lb) lean braising
     lamb, thinly sliced
2 teaspoons dried mint

450 g (1 lb) new potatoes,
     scrubbed and thinly sliced
125 g (5 oz) green beans or
     mangetout
2 tablespoons fresh parsley,
     chopped

Lay out the aubergine slices and cover each with salt. Leave for 30 minutes, then rinse and drain. Heat the oil in a pan and fry the lamb with the mint for 7-10 minutes. Remove the lamb and set aside. Add the potatoes to the pan and sauté for about 5 minutes. Add the beans or mangetout and aubergine, and cook for another 2-3 minutes. Return the lamb and cook for another 5 minutes. Serve garnished with parsley.

RECIPES

Apricot Lamb Pilaf

Serves 4; 425 calories per serving

450 g (1 lb) lean neck of lamb
1 tablespoon corn or sunflower oil
2 medium onions, finely chopped
Salt and black pepper to taste

¼ teaspoon cinnamon
¼ teaspoon allspice
¼ teaspoon nutmeg
2 tablespoons seedless raisins
175 g (6 oz) dried apricots
350 g (12 oz) long-grain rice

Trim visible fat from lamb and cut into 2.5 cm (1 inch) cubes. Heat the oil in a casserole and sauté the lamb gently for 10 minutes. Add the onions and stir-cook for a further 5-10 minutes. Add the salt, pepper and spices, raisins and apricots and sauté for 2-3 minutes. Cover with cold water, bring to the boil and simmer under cover for 80-90 minutes until lamb is tender. Boil rice in lightly salted water until nearly done (about 10 minutes), and drain. Add to the centre of the lamb and sauce, and spoon the sauce over it. Cover and cook in a moderate oven 180°C/350°F/Gas 4 for a further 15 minutes.

Pork and Prunes

Serves 4; 360 calories per serving

2 lean pork fillets or 4 pork chops
150 ml (5 fl oz) dry white wine
250 ml (8 fl oz) water
1 medium onion, finely chopped

200 g (7 oz) pitted prunes
125 g (5 oz) low-fat natural yoghurt
2 tablespoons redcurrant jelly
Dash of lemon juice
Salt and black pepper to taste

RECIPES

Remove visible fat from pork and slice into 2.5 cm (1 in) strips. Brown in a non-stick frying pan. Add the wine, water and onion. Cover and simmer for 15-20 minutes. Add the prunes, simmer for a further 10 minutes. Stir in the yoghurt, redcurrant jelly, lemon juice and seasoning. Serve with new potatoes (not included in calorie count) and green salad.

Bacon and Cauliflower Cheese Bake

Serves 4; 300 calories per serving

2 small cauliflowers
175 g (6 oz) green beans
4 slices of lean bacon
25 g (1 oz) low-fat spread
25 g (1 oz) plain flour
350 ml (12 fl oz) sem-
   skimmed milk

100 g (4 oz) low-fat Cheddar-
   type cheese, grated
Salt and pepper to taste
50 g (2 oz) breadcrumbs

Cut the cauliflowers into florets and slice the beans into short lengths. Boil them in slightly salted water until just tender. Drain and put into four small gratin dishes. Grill the bacon until crisp, chop it and scatter over the vegetables. Melt the low-fat spread in a saucepan, add the flour and cook for a minute or so. Add the milk, two-thirds of the grated cheese and seasoning and stir until the cheese melts. Pour on to the vegetables, scatter over the remaining third of grated cheese and breadcrumbs, and grill or bake until brown.

RECIPES

French Chicken Casserole

Serves 4; 300 calories per serving

1 tablespoon corn or olive oil
4 medium-sized chicken
  breasts, skinned
2 medium leeks, sliced
2 medium carrots, sliced
8 small onions or shallots
150 ml (¼ pint) chicken stock
1 tablespoon flour
300 ml (½ pint) semi-skimmed
  milk

150 ml (¼ pint) dry white
  wine (or more chicken
  stock)
Sprinkling of thyme
Salt and black pepper to taste
2 tablespoons French
  mustard, preferably Dijon
Chopped fresh chives or
  parsley, to garnish

Heat the oil in a flameproof casserole and gently fry the breasts until golden. Remove and set aside. Stir-fry the leeks, carrots and onions for 2-3 minutes. Pour half the stock into a cup and stir in the flour to make a paste. Add this to the casserole and stir well. Add the rest of the stock, milk and wine, and bring to the boil, stirring. Add the chicken, thyme and seasoning. Cover and simmer for 30 minutes. Finally, stir in the mustard and serve garnished with chives or parsley.

Stir-fried Chicken and Mixed Vegetables

Serves 4; 225 calories per serving

4 x 250 g (9 oz) chicken
  thighs
1 tablespoon sunflower oil
225 g (8 oz) sliced runner
  beans (or mangetout)
3 tablespoons water

50 g (2 oz) sliced mushrooms
100 g (4 oz) beansprouts
¼ teaspoon allspice
Salt and black pepper to taste
2 tablespoons finely chopped
  fresh parsley

RECIPES

Remove skin from the chicken thighs and slice into small chunks. Heat the oil in a wok or stir-fry pan. Stir-fry chicken for 5-10 minutes until cooked. Add beans and water and stir for 5-10 minutes until tender but still crunchy. Add the mushrooms, beansprouts, allspice and seasoning, and stir for a few more minutes. Sprinkle on parsley and serve.

Fish with Peppers

Serves 4; 220 calories per serving

2 lemons
450 g (1 lb) any white fish, in
    4 portions
2 tablespoons sunflower,
    corn or olive oil
2 cloves garlic, crushed
2 medium onions, sliced

400 g (14 oz) can chopped
    tomatoes
1 green pepper, de-seeded
    and sliced
1 red pepper, de-seeded and
    sliced
Chopped fresh parsley

Squeeze the juice from one of the lemons over the fish and leave to marinate. Heat the oil in a large pan and gently fry the garlic and onions until softened. Add the tomatoes and peppers, and simmer for 15 minutes. Place the fish in the pan and spoon the sauce over it Thinly slice the remaining lemon and arrange over the fish. Cook for 15-20 minutes, and serve with new potatoes (not in calorie count), brushed with oil and baked in an ovenproof pot. Garnish with parsley.

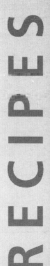

Tuna and Egg Salad

Serves 4; 300 calories per serving (including roll)

2 small lettuce heads
100 g (4 oz) lightly cooked
green beans
200 g (7 oz) new potatoes,
boiled or baked
4 medium tomatoes
8 spring onions
50 g (2 oz) watercress

400 g (14 oz) tuna, canned in
brine
8 tablespoons low-fat French
dressing
2 hard-boiled eggs (size 3),
quartered
8-12 black olives

Break the lettuce into pieces in a large salad bowl.Chop in the beans, potatoes, tomatoes, spring onions and watercress. Add the tuna and dressing. Toss and thoroughly mix the salad, garnish with the eggs and olives, and serve with a wholemeal bread roll.

Prawn and Mushroom Risotto

Serves 4; 400 calories per serving

275 g (10 oz) risotto rice
1 tablespoon, sunflower or
olive oil
1 medium onion, finely
chopped
450 g (1 lb) mushrooms,
sliced
1 clove garlic, crushed

225 g (8 oz) peeled prawns
1 green pepper, de-seeded
and diced
600 ml (1 pint) chicken stock
1 teaspoon dried oregano
Salt and black pepper to taste
2 tablespoons Parmesan or
Cheddar, grated

RECIPES

Cook the rice in boiling lightly salted water for 10 minutes. Heat the oil in a large pan and gently fry the onion until golden. Add the mushrooms and garlic and stir-fry for 2 minutes. Add the prawns and green pepper and stir-fry for a further 2 minutes. Add the stock and oregano and stir. Drain the rice well and add to the mixture in the pan, stirring all the time. Cover and simmer for 10 minutes. Check that the rice is soft and, if the mixture is too liquid, stir-cook without the lid. Season to taste, sprinkle with the cheese and serve.

Worcester Salmon Bake

Serves 4, 350 calories per serving

4 x 175 g (6 oz) salmon
steaks
4 tablespoons reduced-calorie
mayonnaise
1 teaspoon Worcester sauce

4 tablespoons Parmesan,
grated
4 tablespoons snipped fresh
chives

Pre-heat the oven to 220°C/425°F/Gas 7. Place the salmon steaks on a non-stick baking tray. Mix the mayonnaise, Worcester sauce, Parmesan and chives, and spread the mixture on the salmon. Bake for 15 minutes, and serve with a salad from the allowance.

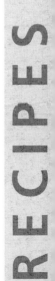

Crab Noodle Stir-Fry

Serves 4; 340 calories per serving

250 g (9 oz) egg noodles
15 ml (1 tablespoon) corn or
sunflower oil
1 bunch spring onions, sliced
lengthwise
2.5 cm (1 in) piece root
ginger, chopped
1 clove garlic, crushed

225 g (8 oz) mangetout,
trimmed
200 g (7 oz) crab sticks, sliced
lengthwise
3 tablespoons light soy sauce
2 level tablespoons cornflour
150 ml (¼ pint) fish or chicken
stock

Cook the noodles in lightly salted boiling water. Meanwhile, heat the oil in a wok or large pan. Add the spring onions, ginger, garlic and mangetout, and stir-fry for 3 minutes. Add the crab sticks and stir-fry for a further 2 minutes. In a bowl, mix the soy sauce into the cornflour and stir in the stock. Add this mixture to the wok or pan, bring to the boil, stirring continuously. Simmer for 2 minutes. Drain the noodles and spread them on a warmed serving dish. Top with the stir-fry and serve.

Tuna Tagliatelle

Serves 4; 450 calories per serving

350 g (12 oz) tagliatelle
175 g (6 oz) can tuna (in
brine, drained)
200 g (7 oz) natural fromage
frais

½ teaspoon caster sugar
Salt and black pepper to taste
25 g (1 oz) half-fat Cheddar
cheese, grated
40 g (1½ oz) breadcrumbs

RECIPES

Cook the pasta in lightly salted water. Meanwhile, flake the tuna into a bowl and thoroughly mix with the fromage frais, sugar and seasoning to taste. Drain the pasta, mix with the tuna mixture and transfer to a warm ovenproof dish. Mix the cheese with the breadcrumbs and sprinkle over the tuna pasta. Grill for a few minutes until brown. Serve with green salad from allowance.

Cod, Leek and Potato Bake

Serves 4; 400 calories per serving

750 g (1¾ lb) potatoes
1 large leek, sliced
300 ml (½ pint) skimmed milk
I tablespoon chopped fresh
    (or dried) parsley
4 teaspoons margarine
50 g (2 oz) plain flour

Salt and black pepper to taste
675 g (1½ lb) cod (or
    haddock), boned, cut into
    chunks
1 egg white
1 tablespoon milk

Boil the potatoes in lightly salted water for about three minutes. Meanwhile, cook the leek in the same way for about 10 minutes. Drain the potatoes and leek, reserving the liquor. Slice the potatoes. Add the skimmed milk and parsley to the liquor. Melt 3 teaspoons of the margarine in a saucepan, add the flour, and cook gently for a minute. Slowly add the milk and parsley mixture, stirring well. Season to taste. Pre-heat the oven to 190°C/375°F/Gas 5. Use the remaining margarine to grease an ovenproof dish, and place the cod in it. Scatter the leeks on top, and cover with the parsley sauce. Arrange the sliced potatoes on top. Paint with a mixture of egg white and milk. Bake for 25-30 minutes.

Vegetable Casserole with Dumplings Ⓥ

Serves 4; 350 calories per serving

Dumplings:
100 g (4 oz) self-raising flour
1 teaspoon ground coriander
Pinch of salt
2 tablespoons pure sunflower
    margarine

Casserole:
2 tablespoons pure sunflower
    oil
1 large carrot, sliced
2 celery sticks, sliced

1 medium leek, sliced
75 g (3 oz) small onions,
    quartered
225 g (8 oz) parsnips, diced
1.2 litres (2 pints) vegetable
    stock
25 g (1 oz) lentils
400 g (14 oz) canned
    chickpeas, drained
225 g (8 oz) cauliflower,
    broken up
Salt and black pepper to taste

Shake the flour into a large bowl, add the coriander and a pinch of salt, and mix well. Blend in the margarine until the mixture is broken up. Add enough cold water to turn it into a soft dough. Make this into eight dumplings. Heat the oil in a large saucepan and lightly sauté the carrot, celery, leek, onions and parsnips for a few minutes. Add the stock, with the lentils and chick peas. Bring to the boil, cover and simmer for 20 minutes. Then add the cauliflower florets and dumplings, cover and simmer for another 20 minutes. Season with salt and black pepper, and serve allowing two dumplings each.

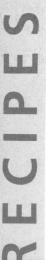

RECIPES

Fish Curry

Serves 4; 250 calories per serving.

750 g (1¾ lb) white fish (cod, haddock) cut into strips
1½ tablespoons oil
1 cm (½ in) fresh root ginger, peeled and sliced
1 clove garlic, sliced
1 large onion, sliced
1 red pepper, de-seeded, cut into strips
1 green chilli (optional), de-seeded and chopped
1 teaspoon ground cumin
1 teaspoon ground coriander
1 teaspoon ground turmeric
Salt and black pepper to taste
125 g (4 oz) curd cheese
Fresh mint, finely chopped

Heat the oil in a pan and gently fry the fish with the ginger and garlic for a few minutes. Set aside the contents of the pan. Add to the pan the onion, pepper and chilli, gently softening without browning. Add the spices and cook for another 2-3 minutes. Return the fish mixture to the pan and half-cover with water. Bring to the boil, season, cover and simmer for 10 minutes. Meanwhile, beat the cheese with a little water, and add to the pan. Bring back to the boil. Serve garnished with the mint.

RECIPES

Tuna and Vegetable Lasagne

Serves 4; 440 calories per serving

2 teaspoons oil
1 medium onion, chopped
2 garlic cloves, crushed
1 large leek, thinly sliced
400 g (14 oz) can chopped
   tomatoes
2 tablespoons tomato purée
2 medium courgettes, thinly
   sliced
1 teaspoon dried oregano
Salt and black pepper to taste
225 g (8 oz) can tuna (in
   brine, drained)

6 x 100 g (4 oz) pre-cooked
   lasagne sheets
100 g (4 oz) mature Cheddar,
   grated

Sauce:
4 teaspoons margarine
25 g (1 oz) plain flour
300 ml (½ pint) skimmed milk
1 teaspoon English made-up
   mustard (optional)

Heat the oil in a large pan and gently fry the onion, garlic and leek for about 5 minutes. Stir in the tomatoes, tomato purée, courgettes, oregano and seasoning. Bring to the boil, cover and simmer for about 15 minutes. Meanwhile, in a smaller pan, melt the margarine, stir in the flour and cook for 1 minute. Slowly whisk in the milk until the sauce thickens. Remove from the heat and stir in the mustard and seasoning. Pre-heat the oven to 190 °C/375° F/Gas 5. Flake the tuna and stir it into the vegetable mixture. Spoon half this mixture into an ovenproof baking dish and cover with three lasagne sheets. Top with half of the sauce and sprinkle with half of the cheese. Then repeat this sequence with the remaining mixture, sheets, sauce and cheese. Bake for about 30 minutes until just turning brown.

RECIPES

Pears in Wine Sauce

Serves 4; 75 calories per serving

4 pears
300 ml (½ pint) medium
   sweet red wine
300 ml (½ pint) water
1 bay leaf

4 cloves
Rind of 1 orange, grated
1 tablespoon ginger wine (or
   sweet sherry)

Peel the pears and place in a saucepan with the wine and water, bay leaf, cloves and orange rind. Bring to the boil, cover and simmer for about 1½ hours. Remove the pears and place each in a small serving bowl. Boil the remaining liquid rapidly to reduce it by half. Remove from the heat, stir in the ginger wine and pour this sauce over the pears to serve.

Summer Pudding

Serves 4; 170 calories per serving

675 g (1½ lb) assorted
   summer fruits –
   blackcurrants, redcurrants,
   blackberries, strawberries,
   raspberries

25 g (1 oz) soft brown sugar
5 x medium slices white
   bread, without crusts

Cook the fruit with the sugar and 2 tablespoons water until juicy and tender, stirring very gently without mashing. Cut the bread into strips and use most of them to line a small (800 ml/1½ pint) pudding basin. Pour the cooked fruit into the basin, reserving 2 tablespoons juice for decoration. Cover with remaining bread strips. Put a saucer on the top, and weight it down. When cool, put in the fridge and leave for 8 hours or overnight to allow the juice to seep through the bread. Invert carefully on to a plate to serve, and pour the remaining juice over the top.

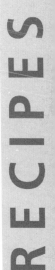

RECIPES

Strawberry Parfait

Serves 4; 160 calories per serving

225 g (8 oz) strawberries
200 ml (7 fl oz) low-fat
strawberry yoghurt
200 ml (7 fl oz) half-fat single
cream

2 egg whites (size 3)
40 g (1½oz) caster sugar

To decorate
4 large fresh strawberries

Blend the strawberries in a blender until smooth. Add the yoghurt and cream, continue blending. Pour into a bowl. In another bowl, whisk the egg whites and caster sugar into a stiff mixture, and fold into the strawberry mixture. Pour this mixture into a plastic freezing tray and chill for 2-3 hours. Mash with a fork and freeze until firm. Thaw slightly before serving with a scoop. Decorate with sliced fresh strawberries.

Spicy Oranges

Serves 4; 100 calories per serving

125 ml (4 fl oz) red wine
4 tablespoons water
2 tablespoons sugar
2 slices lemon

½ cinnamon stick
2 cloves
4 oranges, peeled, pipped
and sliced

Put all ingredients except the oranges into a saucepan and bring to the boil. Continue boiling rapidly until the liquid is reduced by about half. Pour over the orange slices and serve.

RECIPES

Winter Fruit Flan

Serves 4; 180 calories per serving

Base:
75 g (3 oz) wholemeal flour
Pinch salt
⅓ teaspoon baking powder
40 g (1½ oz) margarine
1 teaspoon grated orange
   rind
2 tablespoons water

Filling:
3 medium-sized apples,
   peeled, cored and chopped

175 g (6 oz) apricots, halved
   and stoned
2 small oranges, peeled,
   pipped and sliced,
   reserving a little juice

Glaze:
1½ teaspoons clear honey
2 teaspoons apple juice
   concentrate

Mix the flour, salt and baking powder in a bowl. Rub in the margarine throroughly. Add the orange rind and water. Mix to a soft dough. Knead and roll out to form the flan case in a lightly greased flan tin. Bake in a pre-heated moderate oven, 200°C/400°F/Gas 6 for 5 minutes. Place the apples, apricots and reserved orange juice in a pan, cover and cook for 10 minutes. Purée the mixture in a blender and fill the flan case. Cover with the orange slices. Bake for 20 minutes. Meanwhile, mix the honey and concentrated apple juice. When the flan is done, cool slightly and brush with the honey glaze. Serve warm.

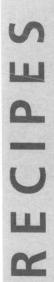

RECIPES

Crunchy Nectarines

Serves 4; 150 calories per serving

50 g (2 oz) oatmeal
50 g (2 oz) chopped walnuts
   or hazelnuts
1 teaspoon orange rind, grated

3 nectarines, peeled, pipped
   and sliced
Juice of 1 orange

Toast the oatmeal in a pre-heated oven 180°C/350°F/Gas 4 for 10 minutes. Cool and mix with nuts and orange rind. Place half the nectarines in a lightly greased flan tin and sprinkle half the crunchy mixture over them. Place the remaining nectarines on top of that and cover with the remaining crunchy mixture. Thoroughly soak the top crunchy layer with the orange juice, using more if necessary. Return to the oven and bake for 30 minutes. Serve warm.

Lemon Sponge Pudding

Serves 4; 250 calories per serving

1 tablespoon soft margarine
25 g (1 oz) brown sugar
5 tablespoons self-raising
   flour

Juice of 1 lemon
Rind of 1 lemon, grated
250 ml (8 fl oz) skimmed milk
1 egg white

Blend the margarine, sugar, flour, lemon juice and rind in a bowl. Stir in the milk. Beat the egg white until stiff and fold into the mixture. Pour into a lightly greased baking dish and bake in a pre-heated oven 180°C/350°F/Gas 4 until just beginning to brown.

RECIPES

Spicy Compote

Serves 4; 150 calories per serving

225 g (8 oz) mixed dried fruit
(such as apricots, prunes,
apples, peaches)

8 cloves
5 cm (2 inch) cinnamon stick
¼ teaspoon grated nutmeg

Cover the dried fruit with water and soak overnight. Place in a pan with the soaking liquid and spices. Bring to the boil, cover and simmer for 45 minutes. Serve hot.

Fruity Fool

Serves 4; 100 calories per serving

225 g (8 oz) fresh or frozen
strawberries, raspberries,
or blackberries
Rind of ½ lemon, grated
Juice of ½ lemon

225 g (8 oz) low-fat natural
fromage frais
Low-calorie granulated
sweetener to taste
4 tablespoons whipped cream

Reserve a few berries for decoration and purée the rest with the rind and juice. Sieve to remove pips and bits. Return to blender, add the fromage frais and sweetener, and blend until mixed. Spoon into four glasses, chill and serve topped with cream and whole berries.

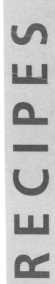

RECIPES

chapter 11

The Body-clock Exercise Programme

Next time you stand naked before the mirror, remind yourself that just beneath those fulsome bulges and ample contours are some of your dearest friends in your quest for the new slim you – your muscles.

While it is certainly true that a sensible low-fat diet is the single most effective way of losing weight, don't forget that it's really only part of the weaponry you can muster in your battle of the bulge.

The other vital element is exercise, or, if the very word fills you with dread, a more active lifestyle.

Diet and exercise are like two sides of the same coin – any slimming programme worthy of the name has to include both because they each can do so much to enhance one another.

And once you've reached your target weight, a more active lifestyle combined with sensible low-fat eating will help to keep you there.

Don't believe those clever-clogs who tell you that exercise is a waste of time and effort as far as slimming is concerned. They're wrong.

And don't believe those languid types who say you have to work out for an hour for every slice of buttered toast you consume. They're wrong too.

There's much more to exercise than just the extra calories you burn while you're doing it. There are other much more subtle effects – particularly for women – and very particularly for women who find dieting a struggle at certain times of the month.

So, don't knock the active life – check it out. Here are just a few benefits you may not be aware of...

Did you know?...
- *regular exercise can help you break through your slimming plateaus*
- *exercise reduces your appetite (it does NOT make you hungry)*
- *exercise can help you to beat food cravings*
- *regular exercise boosts your basal metabolic rate – even at rest*
- *regular exercise can lift your mood*
- *regular exercise can help fend off PMS symptoms*

... and a reminder of the benefits you are probably already aware of:

Regular exercise can...
- *tone and tighten sagging contours*
- *help you to keep supple*
- *help lift depression*
- *improve your sleep*
- *help beat stress*
- *build stronger bones – helping you to avoid osteoporosis (loss of bone strength) in later life*
- *help to keep your blood pressure down*
- *help to protect you against heart disease*

...and, in many ways, the most important benefit of all (and one which only those who have experienced it will truly understand)...

- *Regular exercise can really help you feel good about yourself*

...which, let's face it, is more than half the battle when you are trying to be positive about losing weight and getting back in shape.

Too good to be true?
Is all this just health freaks' hype? Or fitness fanatics' fantasy?

Not a bit of it. Each one of these claims is backed up by solid scientific evidence. And they're all there waiting for you to take advantage of.

So, don't just sit there – get moving!

Excuses, excuses...

You have probably got a long string of very good reasons for not exercising regularly. Here are some of the likeliest:

'I loathe the very word "exercise" and all it stands for'

Okay, look at it another way. Instead, simply think of yourself as being a little more physically active. You don't have to put on all the gear and join an exercise class if you don't want to. You don't have to leap about like a mad thing if you would rather not. All I am saying is that you can gain many of the benefits of exercise by finding ordinary everyday ways of being just that little bit more active.

So, for instance, instead of standing in a lift to go up one or two floors, do something crazy – walk up the stairs!

Instead of stepping on to the escalator and letting yourself be carried – climb up in half the time.

Instead of taking the bus all the way to the shops or to work – get off a stop or two earlier and walk the rest of the way.

Instead of leaving the kids to just droop about the place – chase them round the garden or the local park.

There are loads of ways of being more active without 'exercising' in the grim or off-putting sense of the word. The only barrier is in your mind.

'I haven't got the time'

Of course you haven't. Whether it is the demands of the family, the job, or whatever, your time is not your own. There's not a spare minute in the day. You are busy flat out from dawn till dusk. No, really, honest, it is true.

But is it? Are you absolutely sure there are not even a few moments when you could be a little more active? Couldn't you not just shift one or two things around to make time for exercise? Just 15 minutes a day could make a huge difference. Or 30 minutes, several times a week.

Look at the examples I have just given of ways of making your everyday life more active. Surely you can build on these a little day by day.

And why not get up 15 minutes earlier each day to make time for a fitness session?

Or, set aside part of your lunch-break for a brisk walk?

'I'm too embarrassed'

Many women feel like this – often because they regard themselves as too fat or ungainly or out of condition. They picture themselves being pitied by serried ranks of lithe, lissom nymphets in designer leotards. The prospect is just too awful to contemplate.

But it doesn't have to be like that – and you don't have to feel like that.

For one thing, you don't have to join a class or appear 'in public'. You can easily get in shape in the privacy of your own home. The Body-clock Exercise Programme will show you how.

Second, you don't have to wear a skimpy top or shorts to exercise. Any light loose clothing will do, as long as you can perspire with ease. And let's not forget that walking, one of the best forms of exercise there is for building up your calorie-burning metabolic rate, can be done wearing your ordinary everyday clothes.

And third, there is probably an exercise class near you that is specially aimed at overweight women, so that you and your fellow slimmers can all get over your embarrassment together.

'I'm too unfit – it would kill me'

Whilst there are certainly some people who should seek their doctor's advice before taking up exercise (see page 144), simply being unfit, even very unfit, is no excuse for inactivity.

In fact, you are the very type of person who has most to gain from being active.

As long as you start gently and build up gradually, week by week, never pushing yourself too hard, and always staying within the limits of what is comfortable for you, you should find that your fitness steadily improves and you can do more and more without feeling that it's all too much like hard work.

Athletes call this the 'training effect'. Your body responds to the demands made of it. It becomes stronger, more supple, and better able to cope with activities that previously would have left you a panting, aching wreck.

The less fit you are to start with, the more rapidly and easily you will feel the benefits.

The three 'S-Factors'

Apart from all the benefits I have just listed, whenever you exercise regularly, there are three direct effects on your level of fitness:

- *you improve your Stamina*
- *you build up your Strength*
- *you increase your Suppleness*

These are known as the three S-Factors, and each is important for all round fitness.

Stamina is staying power – the ability to keep going without collapsing in a breathless heap. The best activities for developing stamina are those that make you puffed, that demand oxygen – hence the term 'aerobic' exercise. You probably think of 'aerobics' as those energetic exercises people do in classes or to a video at home. But any activity that makes you a little breathless is aerobic and is good for building stamina. So, brisk walking, swimming, cycling, skipping, climbing stairs, running, disco dancing – all are excellent aerobic activities – and all are great for burning calories.

Strength is just that – the power to push and shove, to lift and carry. It means not only strong muscles, but also strong tendons, ligaments and, last but not least, bones. The stronger your bones are now, the less likely you are to be at risk later on from the osteoporosis that affects so many women after the menopause. And, right now, strength is very helpful for shopping, housework and coping with small children. Toning exercises improve strength. And activities for building strength are those that involve ... yes, you guessed it ... pushing, shoving, lifting and carrying.

Suppleness is flexibility – the ability to move your back and joints through their full range without getting stiff or stuck. When you are truly supple you feel wonderfully loose-limbed and springy. People often say they're 'too stiff to exercise'. That's crazy! They're the very people who would soon feel the difference with just a few minutes of stretching exercises each morning. I do mine while I'm waiting for the hot tap to warm up!

Of course, most popular activities do something to improve all three of these 'S-Factors', as the chart opposite shows and you can gain best all round benefit by choosing a mixture of different activities.

Here are the S-Factor and calorie-burning rates for a wide range of work and play activities.

Activity	Stamina	Strength	Suppleness	Calories
AEROBIC CLASS	●●●	●●●	●●●	60
BADMINTON	●●○	●●○	●●●	65
BEDMAKING	●○○	●○○	●●○	40
BODY CONDITIONING	●●○	●●●	●●○	45
CLEANING HOUSE	●○○	●●○	●●○	40
COOKING	●○○	●○○	●○○	30
CYCLING (EASY)	●○○	●●○	●○○	40
CYCLING (HARD)	●●●	●●●	●○○	70
DANCING (BALLROOM)	●○○	●○○	●●○	35
DANCING (DISCO)	●●●	●●○	●●○	65
DRIVING A CAR	○○○	○○○	○○○	20
DUSTING	●○○	●○○	●○○	20
EATING	○○○	○○○	○○○	15
GARDENING (DIG)	●●○	●●●	●○○	70
GARDENING (HAND MOW)	●●●	●●○	●○○	70
GARDENING (WEED)	●○○	●○○	●●○	35
GOLF	●●○	●●○	●●○	55
GYMNASTICS	●●○	●●●	●●●	50
GYM WORKOUT	●●●	●●●	●●●	85
HOCKEY	●●●	●●○	●○○	85
HOME DECORATING	●○○	●●○	●●○	30
HORSE RIDING	●○○	●●○	●○○	40
ICE SKATING	●●○	●●○	●●○	50
IRONING	●○○	●○○	●○○	20
JOGGING	●●●	●●○	●○○	80
JUDO	●○○	●●●	●●○	40
KNITTING	○○○	○○○	○○○	15
LYING AT EASE	○○○	○○○	○○○	15
MOPPING THE FLOOR	●○○	●○○	●●○	40
NETBALL	●●○	●●○	●●●	70
PIANO PLAYING	○○○	○○○	●○○	25
ROCK CLIMBING	●●○	●●●	●●○	40
ROLLER SKATING	●●○	●●●	●○○	50
RUNNING (10 MINS/MILE)	●●●	●●○	●○○	120
SEWING (MACHINE)	○○○	○○○	○○○	25
SHOPPING	●○○	●○○	●○○	40
SITTING	○○○	○○○	○○○	15
SKIING	●●○	●●●	●●○	65
SKIPPING	●●●	●●○	●○○	105
SLEEPING	○○○	○○○	○○○	10
SQUASH	●●●	●●●	●●●	120
STAIR CLIMBING	●●●	●●●	●○○	110
STANDING STILL	○○○	●○○	○○○	15
STRETCH CLASSES	●○○	●○○	●●●	30
SWEEPING	●○○	●○○	●●○	30
SWIMMING (HARD)	●●●	●●●	●●●	100
TABLE TENNIS	●●○	●●○	●●●	45
TENNIS	●●○	●●○	●●●	60
TYPING	○○○	○○○	○○○	20
VACUUM CLEANING	●○○	●●○	●●○	40
VOLLEYBALL	●●○	●●○	●●●	50
WALKING (STROLLING)	●○○	●●○	●○○	40
WALKING (BRISKLY)	●●●	●●○	●○○	60
WASHING DISHES	○○○	○○○	●○○	20
WEIGHT TRAINING	●●●	●●●	●●○	60
YOGA	●○○	●○○	●○○	30
YOMPING (JOG/WALK)	●●●	●●●	●○○	70

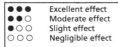

●●●	Excellent effect
●●○	Moderate effect
●○○	Slight effect
○○○	Negligible effect

NOTE: Calorie expenditure is for 10 minutes of typical continuous activity by a woman of average height who is 6kg (14lb) overweight. If you have more than this to lose, you will burn up calories faster.

...and two more of my own...

Here are two extra 'S-Factors' that exercise can give you. I've added these myself because I believe they are particularly important for slimmers.

'**Sparkle**' is that indefinable radiance that active people feel. It shows in their bright eyes and healthy glow, the absence of 'worry-lines', the zest for life. 'Sparkle' can make you feel positive about yourself, even in times of stress and grimness. 'Sparkle' can help you keep to your diet instead of giving up at the first hurdle.

'**Spin**' – no, nothing to do with the ability to twirl on your toes! By 'spin' I mean the quickness of your body chemistry when you are at rest – in other words your 'tickover' speed or basal metabolic rate. Imagine there is a sort of flywheel spinning away inside you, powering all those body processes that are happening all the time, even when you are resting. The faster it spins, the more calories it uses up. So, the more you can do to increase your flywheel 'spin', the easier it will be to lose weight and maintain slimness.

The speed of your flywheel depends greatly on how much lean tissue you have – in other words, muscle. Muscle has a higher metabolic rate than bodyfat, even when it's doing nothing. Remember the old saying: 'Inside every fat woman is a thin one trying to get out'? Well, if you can make your 'thin woman' a bit more muscular, with regular aerobic activities and toning exercises, you can do quite a lot to boost your 'spin'.

Any activity that scores two or three stars in the 'Stamina' or 'Strength' column of the chart will help. But it's not just a matter of how vigorous the exercise is – it's also for how long and how frequently you do it. So, for example, although brisk walking is not particularly vigorous – if you do it for long enough and often enough, it can really get that flywheel spinning – perhaps more than a once-weekly workout!

How much? How often?

The answer is: as much as you can manage comfortably and without disrupting your life.

But, to put a figure on it, if you can have at least an hour's-worth of moderately vigorous activity a week – say, two x 30-minute sessions, three x 20-minute sessions, four x 15-minute sessions, or even six x 10-minute sessions of an activity that gets you about as puffed as brisk walking – that would make a very useful contribution to all five 'S-Factors' and your weight control programme.

The latest 'official' recommendation from experts in the USA is 30 minutes a day of moderate activity like this – not necessarily all in one go. If you can manage that, so much the better for your 'sparkle' and 'spin'!

Exercise and plateau-busting

How often have you found yourself up against a rock solid plateau, with your scales absolutely point-blank refusing to go any lower even though you are being really good about your diet and doing all the right things?

The reason this happens is because, in your enthusiasm to lose weight fast, the low calorie content of your diet has triggered the dreaded 'famine response'. Some monitoring centre deep in your brain has twigged what is happening, rung the alarm, and put the brakes on your 'flywheel' – slowing down your metabolism. So your body doesn't burn so many calories, and you stop losing weight. A thoroughly frustrating and depressing state of affairs.

But, fortunately, there is an answer.

You must take the heat out of the situation by easing up a little on your diet. This means adding about 250 calories to your daily intake (for example, by converting from Plan 1000 to Plan 1250) to lull the monitoring centre into a false sense of security, so that it releases the brakes on your flywheel and allows the metabolism to speed up again.

Unfortunately this adjustment can take about two weeks. So, to bust the plateau sooner, boost your exercise.

By putting extra time and effort into your exercise programme at this critical juncture, you can put extra 'spin'-power into your metabolism straight away. If all goes according to plan, you should be able to restart the weight-loss despite the extra calories.

Exercise and your biorhythms

But what about exercise as far as your menstrual cycle and other biorhythms are concerned?

Well, as you might expect, it varies a great deal from woman to woman.

Many women find that moderately vigorous, even very vigorous, exercise helps them not only to cope with their premenstrual symptoms, but also the discomfort or pain of the period itself.

In the week before the period, daily aerobics or other strenuous activity can do wonders to ease the tension, irritability and low mood.

During menstruation itself, running can be wonderfully soothing for the low back pain and pelvic cramps. Skipping is another remedy – all that jumping up and down seems somehow to massage the aching womb and its tender attachments.

Researchers at Australia's Bond University, Queensland, have shown that regular moderately vigorous aerobic exercise (like brisk walking, skipping, swimming, cycling or running) throughout the whole cycle can improve some symptoms of PMS (premenstrual syndrome) – especially the bad moods, lack of concentration, and aches and pains.

The 'sparkle' effect of exercise can help too – admittedly an uphill struggle in the premenstrual phase! – but with enough tonic effect to help many women feel positive about themselves and stick to their diet, to lift their spirits and get rid of pent-up tension and frustration.

The drag factor

But, by contrast, a lot of women feel so dreadful in the second half of their cycle, so utterly lacking in energy or motivation of any sort, so wrung-out and useless, that going through the motions of exercise is just too much to even contemplate. The thought of dragging themselves over to the leisure centre or getting into all the gear would never even enter their heads.

Both reactions are equally normal and natural. Most women feel much less inclined to take exercise in the second half of their cycle than in the first. Enthusiasm, energy, endurance and co-ordination all tend to be at least a little reduced at that time of the month. The best time for physical activity is usually immediately after a period.

Research studies, summarized by Dr C.M. Lebrun of the University of British Columbia, Vancouver, Canada, have shown that, even among top female athletes, about half find that their performance falls away at certain times of the month, usually in their premenstrual phase. About a quarter have noticed a distinct improvement during and immediately after their period.

These findings are backed by physiological studies which indicate that, although women don't seem to get any sweatier or more breathless when they exercise during Phase B or C, they do tend to have a more rapid heartbeat (a sign of decreased tolerance to exercise) and feel that the effort involved is harder than during Phase A.

So, whether or not you feel inclined to keep exercising throughout your cycle will depend very much on how these changes affect your energy and motivation. That, in turn, will depend on how beneficial you feel that exercising is at different times of the month.

Exercise and food craving

Exercise can not only take your mind off food, it can also banish hunger for some while afterwards. Regular exercise boosts the brain's 'pleasure hormones' which can alleviate the craving for sweet things. A number of studies have shown that aerobic exercise during Phase C of the cycle can substantially reduce cravings in some women – which could make all the difference between success or failure with your diet.

Listen to your mind and body

The advantages of keeping moving throughout your cycle, for some slimmers at least, are quite clear, but even so may not be enough to overcome the inertia most women feel in the days before their period.

The answer to the question 'Is it worth it?'must be to give it a try and listen to your mind and body. You will soon know if you feel better or worse. And you will soon discover whether your moods and cravings improve ... or do not.

Body-clock Exercise Guidelines

Once you've decided to become a more active person, you don't necessarily have to embark on a rigidly prescribed exercise or activity 'programme'. You can simply begin by choosing more active ways of doing ordinary everyday things – choosing the 'active option'. Then, week by week, you should do a little more than you're used to, and slowly build up your activity and fitness level. Remember not to push yourself to the point of discomfort. If it hurts in the slightest, you're doing it wrong.

Here are the 'golden rules' for more active living:
- choose the 'active option' whenever you can.
- choose activities you enjoy – go for variety.
- start gently and build up gradually week by week.
- let your body be your guide – if you feel uncomfortable, slow down or stop.
- remember to warm up before vigorous exercise – and cool down after.
- never exercise if you're tired or ill.
- check with your doctor first if you are at all worried about your health.

Three levels of activity
If you do prefer some general guidance about how much time to devote to exercise each week, here are three brief programmes which differ according to the intensity and frequency of effort required. The routines are described on pages 147-150.

If you're very unfit or not used to exercise, it is best to start with the Low Intensity Programme and progress from there. If you are already fairly active you could go straight into either the Medium or High Intensity Programme.

Low Intensity Programme

This is a fairly minimal programme, requiring a home stretch-and-tone session twice a week, and an hour of moderately vigorous 'active options' each week.

Stretch routine – 5 minutes, twice a week
Tone routine – 10 minutes, twice a week
Aerobic activity – 60 minutes' worth of 'active options'
throughout the week

Medium Intensity Programme

This programme is based on a 35-minute session three times a week, or every other day, with one day off. Again the aerobic activity can be split into two or three separate bouts.

Stretch routine – 5 minutes, three times a week
Tone routine – 10 minutes, three times a week
Aerobic activity – 20 minutes, three times a week

High Intensity Programme

This programme involves a total of 45 minutes exercise a day, although the aerobic activity could comprise up to three separate bouts of exercise, each lasting not less than 10 minutes. You are allowed a day off a week if you like.

Stretch routine – 5 minutes, daily
Tone routine – 10 minutes, daily.
Aerobic activity – 30 minutes, daily
(not necessarily all in one session)

What time of day is best?

The answer to that is whenever you can best manage it. But, if you have some choice in the matter, here are a few pointers:

Stretch-and-tone sessions are particularly beneficial first thing in the morning to set you up for the day.

The best time for aerobic activity depends to some extent on whether you are a 'lark' or an 'owl'. Larks usually enjoy exercise more in the early part of the morning or early evening – owls late morning or late afternoon.

Many slimmers find that an aerobic session at their usual 'peak craving time', or just before it, helps to take away the urge to gorge.

Needless to say, to avoid cramps and discomfort you should not take part in vigorous exercise too soon after a meal. Allow an hour or so for your food to go down. But most of these considerations are fairly minor. The important thing is to choose times that suit you best and fit the activity in with all your other commitments. Use your answer to Question 9 on page 47 to help you decide.

Your Monthly Activity Planner

Here are some suggestions as to how to plan your physical activities according to the phase of your monthly cycle.

Phase A activities

This is likely to be your 'all right' phase, and for most women is the best time of the month for fat-burning, aerobic and toning activities.

If you are already fairly fit or active, join the Medium or High Intensity Programme.

If you have never really taken up exercise in an organized or regular way before, this is the best time to start. Take it easy at first, building up week by week. The Low Intensity Programme is recommended for the first month.

Phase B activities

In this part of your cycle you may feel less inclined to exercise, or find it rather more of an effort. But because your metabolic rate is slightly increased in the second half of your cycle, you can afford to ease up a little if you want to.

If you were on the High Intensity Programme, you may prefer to switch to the Medium or even Low Intensity Programme. But by all means carry on with the High Intensity if you are feeling okay. The important thing is to keep up the frequency and duration of the sessions, even if you do not work yourself quite so hard.

Phase C activities

This, for most women, is the least favourite time for exercise, although, as we saw above, aerobic activities in particular can bring real benefits in terms of lifting low spirits, releasing pent-up tension, and reducing hunger and food cravings.

If you do keep yourself moving, it is wise to steer clear of activities requiring perfect co-ordination, particularly if mistakes could be dangerous – gymnastics or rock climbing for example.

If you really don't feel like keeping up your usual activity, try at least to adopt the Low Intensity Programme during this phase, and make as many of those 'active option' changes as you can. And if that's too much effort for you, then at least continue with the twice weekly stretch routine, which only takes about 5 minutes but helps to keep your muscles and joints supple and ready for your next Phase A

Stretch Routine

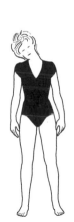
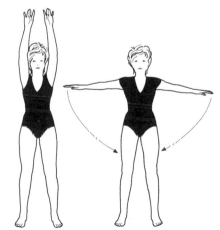

Neck Stretching. Stand, feet apart, arms hanging loose. Tilt your head to one side so that it gently stretches the muscles on the opposite side of your neck. Repeat on the other side. Don't force it. Alternate ten times.

Arm Circling. Stand, feet slightly apart, arms extended straight in front of you, palms down. Raise both arms until directly above you, and, keeping them straight and pushing them as far back as is comfortable, lower them slowly down to your sides, before raising them up again to the starting position. Repeat as a smooth continuous movement ten times.

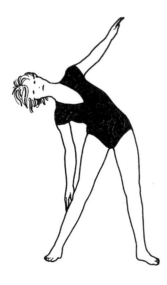

Side Stretching. Stand, feet wide apart, arms straight out to each side, palms down. Keeping your arms in a straight line, tilt the upper half of your body to one side, so that one arm is reaching down your outer thigh and the other is pointing at the ceiling. Tilt as far as is comfortable and return to the upright position. Repeat on the other side, and alternate ten times.

Ham and Calf Stretching. Stand, feet apart, arms hanging loosely. Take a step forward with your left foot, bend your left knee, rest your hands on your left thigh, just above the knee, and transfer your weight to the left leg, keeping your right foot flat on the floor. Feel your hamstrings (back of thigh) and calf stretching. Stretch forward ten times and do the same on the other side.

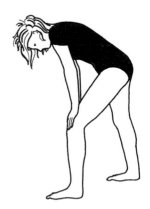

Tone Routine

Press-ups *(for chest, upper arms, and trunk).* Kneel on all fours with your knees slightly apart. Bend your elbows and slowly lower your head and shoulders until your forehead touches the floor. Raise slowly to the horizontal and repeat eight times. As you get stronger, place your hands further forwards until you're eventually doing full straight leg press-ups, with your bottom held up.

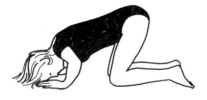

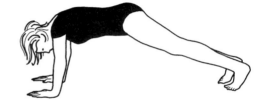

Flank toner *(for hips and outer thighs)*. Lie on your side, with your lower leg slightly bent, your upper leg straight, and your head resting on your hands as a pillow. Raise your upper leg about 45°, keeping your pelvis at right angles to the floor. Hold for a slow count of ten, and relax. Repeat eight times. Turn over and do the same with the other leg.

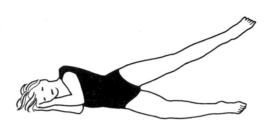

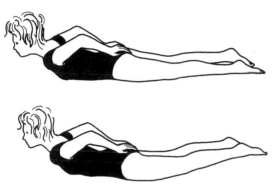

Back toner *(for a firm back and bottom)*. Lie face down, palms on your bottom. Now, imagine a rope under your elbows being lifted by a crane. Keeping your hands on your bottom, push your elbows together and skywards, raising your head and shoulders from the floor and tensing your bottom. Hold for a slow count of ten and relax. Repeat eight times. As you get stronger, raise both legs off the ground at the same time.

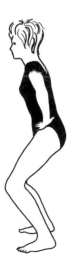

Half Squats *(for bottom and thighs)*. Stand, feet slightly apart, arms on your hips. Bend your knees, sticking your bottom out so that you're half crouching. Hold for a slow count of ten. Repeat eight times. As you get stronger, crouch a little deeper.

Tummy toners *(for a flatter tum)* Lie on your back with your knees half-bent, and your feet flat on the floor. Slowly lift your head and shoulders, sliding your hands down your thighs to touch your kneecaps. Hold for a count of ten. Repeat eight times. As you get stronger, lock your hands behind your head and wedge your feet under a piece of furniture.

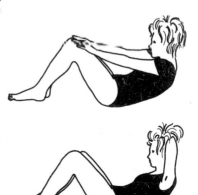

Home Aerobics Routine

This is a simple aerobic routine for you to do at home, to music if you prefer. Remember to let your breathing be your guide. Don't let yourself get more than mildly breathless. Try to keep going with a mixture of activities for at least 20 minutes.

As with any vigorous aerobic exercise, you should warm up first with your stretch routine (and tone routine if you have time). Don't forget to cool down afterwards with a shortened version of your stretch routine to prevent stiffness.

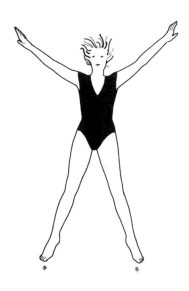

Marching Drum-marjorette-style. Kick your knees high, and really swing those arms. Keep it up for at least five minutes.

Stepping. Using the first or second step of the stairs. Step up and down, one foot following the other. Keep it up for at least five minutes.

Skipping. This is a great exercise if you've got the room for it. And you can challenge yourself to do a certain number of double or triple skips each time. Keep it up for at least five minutes.

'X'-Jumps. Starting with your feet together and arms at your sides, jump to the 'X' position with your feet apart and arms flung out. Jump back again, and repeat, keeping on your toes. Keep it up for at least five minutes.

These are merely suggestions. If you prefer to use a trampoline, exercise bike, rowing machine or whatever, go right ahead!

Anything's good if it gets you moving!

CHAPTER 12

Staying Slim

Hey, look at that! You finally did it! You harnessed the power of your body-clock and biorhythms to shake off all those excess pounds. Perhaps more easily than you thought possible. Or maybe more of a struggle than you ever imagined!

But, anyway, here you are, down to a much better weight. The challenge now is to keep it like that. So, let's look at how you can use the Body-clock StaySlim Plan to avoid the dreaded yo-yo.

Don't throw it all away

The most important thing is NOT to say, 'Right. That's it. Diet's over. Where's the biscuit tin?', before you have even stepped off the scales.

Ending your diet does NOT mean you can simply go back to where you left off, with all your old disastrous eating habits. To stand any chance of keeping your weight off, it is crucial that you continue to be as careful about what you eat, and how much exercise you take, as you were during the slimming process.

In some ways I think it's best not to think in terms of 'coming off your diet' in the sense of abandoning all the principles and rules. Yes, you will have much more flexibility ... and much more food. But you will still need to be just as concerned about the fat and calorie content, just as careful when you shop, cook and serve, and just as clever about using Body-clock methods to cope with monthly mood swings and food cravings. So, in a sense, the diet doesn't really go away – it becomes altered and added to. But its spirit lives on as a guiding hand. It becomes a way of life. An eating plan.

But before you reach that happy state, we have to wean you off it – a slow and painstaking process. For quite a while yet you will still be eating the same balance of foods at the same phases of your cycle as before.

But, the big difference is that you will be eating MORE. Not quite as much as you did before you started the diet, but certainly more than during it.

The trick is to find out just how much more you can eat without putting on fat – a feat which requires some neat juggling with the diet 'extras' and your scales.

The return of the 'phantom fat'

The first shock-horror to be prepared for is the sudden gain of a few pounds within a few days of eating higher-calorie meals. This is the famous 'phantom fat' coming back to haunt you.

Remember, when you first started the diet, how you were gratified to find that you lost maybe two, three or more pounds in the first week? And how your elation turned to disappointment when you discovered that nearly all of this was water? (see page 12).

Well, I did warn you that this 'phantom fat' would return when you stopped the diet (or broke it part way through) – and this is something you will have to make allowances for. Once your body starts receiving a normal maintenance calorie intake, its first reaction is to replenish the glycogen 'instant' energy stores in your liver – a process which requires quite a volume of water. (By the way, it is no good trying to prevent this by not drinking – your system will use internal water and give you a raging thirst!)

So, strictly speaking, you have not quite reached your target weight yet, because you haven't made allowances for those phantom pounds. But not to fret, we can sort that out over the next few weeks, because the trick is to get you off the diet so surreptitiously that you don't notice the phantom pounds creeping back on!

Time it right

The first thing is to get the timing right as far as your menstrual cycle is concerned. So, even though the scales may have hit the magic number, usually in the first half of your cycle, you should continue with the diet as before until your next period, or until you would normally start your next Phase A. You may even find you lose an extra pound or two by then, which will be all to the good.

Now, over the next few cycles, we're gradually going to add more food to your diet, whilst at the same time keeping a watchful eye on your weight for signs of fat re-appearing – not water, which is unavoidable, but the real enemy, fat.

At the same time it's important not to let up on your exercise programme – because if you do you will throw the whole re-adjustment process out of kilter, and we will not know where we are with it.

Yes, I know it all sounds a bit of a drag. Just when you thought you could relax at last, you're now told that there are weeks or months more of being careful. But we have to do it like this if you're going to succeed in making the transition from weight loss to the new stay-slim you.

So, the next few cycles are the re-adjustment stage of your Body-clock StaySlim Plan. We will use these cycles to slowly increase your calorie intake and eventually work out the exact calorie requirements you need to maintain yourself at your slimmer weight.

Here are the cycle-by-cycle instructions for making that transition successfully. Make sure you wait until the start of the next cycle before you change anything.

First re-adjustment cycle
From Day 1 of your Phase A, switch from the slimming plan you are currently on to the plan with an extra 250 calories. For example if you reached your target on Plan 1000, then switch to Plan 1250. Or from Plan 1250 to Plan 1500. If you were on Plan 1500 when you reached your target, simply add an extra 250 calories from the Healthy Xtras 250 list.

Target Slimming Diet	First Re-adjustment Diet
Plan 1000	Plan 1250
Plan 1250	Plan 1500
Plan 1500	Plan 1500 + 250

These extra 250 calories are unlikely to make much difference to your weight, although you should find you don't lose as much as you have been.

Second re-adjustment cycle
In this cycle, we continue to add food to your diet to see what effect it has on your weight. The idea is to find out the most you can take in without putting on real weight (fat as opposed to fluid).

At your next Phase A, move up another 250 calories – from Plan 1250 to Plan 1500, or from Plan 1500 to Plan 1500 plus an item from Healthy Xtras 250, and so on.

Target Slimming Diet	Second Re-adjustment Diet
Plan 1000	Plan 1500
Plan 1250	Plan 1500 + 250
Plan 1500	Plan 1500 + 500

Whoa there!
So far then we have added an average of about 500 calories to the daily quota you were having on the diet, and we should now begin to be a little wary about the possibility of real fat weight gain. It shouldn't happen just yet – the average woman who is moderately active should be able to consume about 2000 calories a day without putting on weight – but nevertheless from now onwards we must tread carefully.

Third re-adjustment cycle
The crucial weighing to watch is the lowest in each cycle – usually the first or second weighing in Phase A. Keep comparing it with the same weighing the previous month.

Providing there is no gain in this monthly weighing, add a further 100 calories to your previous intake, selecting items from the Healthy Xtras 100 list.

Target Slimming Diet	Third Re-adjustment Diet
Plan 1000	Plan 1500 + 100
Plan 1250	Plan 1500 + 250 + 100
Plan 1500	Plan 1500 + 500 + 100

This is the sequence you must now repeat each cycle until you see your weight bob up at that crucial monthly weighing.

For each cycle, add 100 calories – no more (you cannot rush this) – to your intake for the same phase of the previous cycle.

... until that fateful day!

As soon as you find that you have put weight on at the crucial weighing, cut back your daily intake by 200 calories – that is the 100 you have just added, plus another 100. This should hold your weight steady at the next month's crucial weighing. If not, take off another 100.

The intakes that you are left with are your 'permanent' maintenance intakes – in other words, your personalized Body-clock StaySlim Plan.

Let's say, for example, that having been on Plan 1000 when you stopped slimming, you are just embarking on your fourth re-adjustment cycle (Plan 1500 + 200 cals) when the scales give you the bad news. You should immediately drop back to Plan 1500 and, providing this holds your weight steady at the next month's crucial weighing, this becomes your StaySlim Plan.

Head spinning?

If all this sounds incredibly complicated, take it from me that it is not really. You will very quickly get the hang of it in practice.

Maintaining yourself

Now you've worked out your StaySlim Plan in terms of calorie intakes, you can begin the more pleasurable business of translating it into whichever foods or meals you particularly fancy.

So far, you've been juggling with the recipes in the Body-clock Diet and the rather limited list of extras, treats and other bits and pieces. But there's nothing to stop you devising a diet of your very own – still tuned to your cycle phases – using your StaySlim Plan calorie intakes as your guide. You don't have to match the calorie quota exactly every day – a little over or under won't matter.

If you go out for dinner somewhere nice, where the food is wonderful, there's no need to skimp or deny yourself some delectable dish – you can always make up for it over the next few days. The crucial thing is not to consistently eat more than your plan allows. The only circumstance which would permit that would be if you were to become very much more physically active – like joining an Olympic team for instance!

Calories, calories, calories....

Does all this mean you're going to be counting calories for the rest of your life?

No, not if you do not want to.

After all, you've been living with the Body-clock Diet for months now. It has become like an old friend. You know each other so well. The Diet has accommodated all your little ups and downs, and provided comfort in your many moments of need. And you, in turn, have come to understand the Diet's basic principles and its own little weaknesses and excesses. You and the Diet are now an 'item'!

So, you should by now have a pretty shrewd idea of what you can, and what you cannot, eat and roughly how much you can get away with. You probably do not need to count calories 'one by one' any more. But hopefully you will always have a kind of sixth sense about where the little blighters are lurking.

Fat – your arch enemy

An awful lot of them are packed into the fat in your food. If you could only keep close tabs on just one aspect of your daily eating habits, it would have to be the amount of fatty, oily, creamy, buttery or chocolatey things you consume. With almost anything else you can err on the generous side without doing too much damage to your figure – apart perhaps from sugar, which is all too easy to eat far too much of. But even a little more fatty food than you should have, if repeated often enough, will very soon have your weight creeping up again.

Expand your repertoire

The Body-clock Diet has lots of delicious and satisfying recipes – some of which you must know pretty well by now! So, if you have not done so already, now is the time to branch out and try all sorts of other calorie-counted recipes, meal ideas and menus. Scour the magazines and bookstands, raid the library, borrow from friends, try the low-calorie prepared meals from the supermarket – whatever you like – the more variety the better.

Go for balance

As well as variety, the other watchword is 'balance'. The whole idea behind the Body-clock Diet is balance.

- *Balancing your calorie intake to your metabolic rate.*
- *Balancing your physical activity with your lifestyle.*
- *Balancing your carbohydrate and fat intakes with your body chemistry at each phase of your monthly cycle.*
- *Balancing your need to watch your weight with the demands of everyday life.*

Two potential pitfalls

This balance can be all-too-easily upset by so many things – stress, bereavement, redundancy, money worries, emotional torment, a failing relationship. But also by two other very common occurrences – injury and pregnancy.

If you become injured – for example, you sprain your ankle or hurt your back – and have to cut back your exercise programme, remember to cut back your calories proportionally – by about 250 calories a day if you have to stop the High Intensity Programme, about 100 calories a day if you have to stop the Medium Intensity Programme, and 100 calories every *other* day for the Low Intensity Programme.

If you decide to try for a baby, or you find you are pregnant, stop the slimming diet, and eat as much as you like of a healthy balance of foods – but not too many fatty or sugary things. You don't have to 'eat for two'!

When eventually you've had your baby, finished breastfeeding, and your periods have restarted, you can get out your old Body-clock Diet book, blow the dust off it, clutch it to your bosom like the old friend it is, and start all over again!

The search goes on...

Meanwhile, I shall continue to study the links between mood, food and body rhythms, and I would be delighted to hear of your experiences with the Body-clock Diet – good, bad or indifferent. Please write to me c/o BBC Books Editorial Department, BBC Worldwide, Woodlands, 80 Wood Lane, London W12 0TT. Your story could be of great help in my search for better ways to help women cope with the difficulties and frustrations of trying to control their weight without ruining their lives.

All the very best to you – health, happiness and harmony.

Index